Malaria

A Handbook for Health Professionals

malaria
consortium

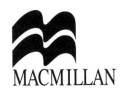

MACMILLAN

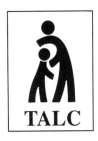

TALC

Macmillan Education
Between Towns Road, Oxford OX4 3PP
A division of Macmillan Publishers Limited
Companies and representatives throughout the world

www.macmillan-africa.com

ISBN: 978-0-333-68916-5

Text © The Malaria Consortium 2007 Design © Macmillan Publishers Limited 2007

First published 2007

Designed by Jim Weaver Design
Typeset by Color & Print Gallery Sdn Bhd, Malaysia
Illustrated by TechType
Cover design by Gary Fielder, AC Design
Cover photographs © Sylvia Meek, except mosquito © Chris Curtis

The authors and publishers would like to thank the following for permission to
reproduce their photographs: The London School of Hygiene & Tropical Medicine pp 15, 16; James Tibenderana pp 65, 117; Daniel Chandramohan p 67; Julia
Mortimer p 144; Tony Wilkes p 146; Chris Curtis p 157; Sylvia Meek for all other
photographs used in this book

The authors and publishers would like to thank the following for permission to
reproduce copyright material: The World Health Organization for a map, tables
and figures on pp 3, 14, 18, 53, 75, 92, 114, 116, 119, 148, 181; Hodder Arnold
for the tables on pp 10 and 23, adapted and reproduced by permission of Hodder Arnold; H. D. Hudson Manufacturing Company for the image on page 156,
courtesy of H. D. Mfg Co., Liverpool School of Tropical Medicine for the table
on p 19, reproduced from the Annals of Tropical Medicine and Parasitology, with
the permission of the Liverpool School of Tropical Medicine

Printed and bound in Malaysia

2014   2013   2012   2011   2010
8   7   6   5   4   3

Contents

Foreword

As early as 500 BC, Empedocle from the city of Agrigento (Italy) noted an association between stagnant water and human disease, and that by environmentally altering the speed of flow of the water a distinct reduction in disease occurred.

Hippocrates distinguished the various types of fever including tertian and quartan and that these fevers were more frequent in Summer and Autumn, where stagnant waters existed, especially following heavy rains in the Spring.

As early as 1883 Dr King in America published a paper giving nineteen reasons why the malaria poison was brought from the marshes by mosquitoes which had bred there and then inoculated it by their bites into human beings – very near but not quite the truth!

During the years that have elapsed between the start of the malaria eradication campaign in 1955 and the publication of this book, there has been a series of changes of strategy from eradication to malaria control; to control of malaria as an integral part of National Primary Health Systems; to a global malaria control strategy to Roll Back Malaria. This shift of strategies has yet to produce significant socio-economic benefit or a significant reduction in morbidity and mortality, particularly in Africa south of the Sahara, where the global burden of malaria is greatest, affecting predominantly children and pregnant women.

Wonder might well be expressed that in spite of all the knowledge of the causative parasite; of the mode of its transmission; of the habits of the vector; of the availability of effective antimalarial drugs (until widespread resistance developed in the 1980s), the results of this knowledge have been disappointing.

Chloroquine resistance was first reported in the 1960s, yet despite the exponential increase that has occurred since then, chloroquine monotherapy has remained until recently the first line treatment for *Plasmodium falciparum* malaria in Africa, despite evidence that it was patently and increasingly failing. Furthermore results of several experimental studies in animals that showed that combination therapy could delay malaria resistance were persistently ignored, as was the established practice of combination therapy for the treatment of tuberculosis and leprosy.

I am confident that the burden of malaria can be reduced with the methods currently in use and the advances in knowledge and novel antimalarials that will become available as a result of the active research that is being undertaken. The adoption of artemisinin-based combination therapy, its acceptability and affordability (hopefully through donor generosity for an initial period of at least five years); the use of long-lasting insecticidal nets; intermittent preventive treatment in pregnancy; intermittent preventive treatment for infants; home management of malaria and the judicious use of artemisinin derivative suppositories are eminently suitable and sustainable interventions.

The training of the private sector is critical bearing in mind that 20–90% of antimalarials sold in seven African countries failed quality testing; and that 11–60% of artesunate sold in the markets of Southeast Asia did not have any active ingredients. The involvement of community based drug distributors and mothers is equally important since over 50% of children with fever are given antimalarials at home and most children in Africa who die from malaria do so at village level, without ever reaching any health facility.

I welcome the publication of this book, the purpose of which is to provide in a concise form the epidemiological, clinical and control aspects of malaria, particularly but not exclusively for district health officers.

The editors as well as the authors of each of the seven chapters have been intimately involved at the 'front line' in the fight against malaria, and their approach is consistently realistic, practical and authoritative. Its publication is timely since decentralisation of health services is occurring in many tropical countries.

Professor H. M. Gilles
Liverpool School of Tropical Medicine

May 2006

Preface

The early 21st century is a critical moment in the fight against malaria. There is at last a set of prevention and treatment methods, which have been shown to work well. There is funding to allow even the most poor and vulnerable people to benefit from these interventions. A key ingredient needed to make the most of this opportunity is a well-informed and committed workforce in every health programme where malaria is a problem.

It is often difficult for health professionals to find comprehensive basic information in the district health programmes where much of the planning and implementation of malaria control takes place. For this reason Macmillan publishers approached the Malaria Consortium to develop a handbook to fill this gap.

This handbook provides accessible and up-to-date information on malaria and its control. After describing the biology of the parasite and mosquito and the epidemiology of the disease, it provides practical advice on diagnosis, treatment and prevention of malaria, control of malaria in pregnancy and planning and managing malaria control programmes.

District health workers can use it as a sourcebook for planning their work, as a reference for implementing and reporting their work, and as a resource for teaching. As well as being packed with facts and methods, it has an extensive glossary for reference.

The handbook was initially developed by the United Kingdom Department for International Development's Malaria Consortium Resource Centre, a project of the London School of Hygiene & Tropical Medicine (LSHTM) and the Liverpool School of Tropical Medicine (LSTM). The different chapters have been written by malaria specialists from LSHTM, LSTM, the Malaria Consortium, Kenya Medical Research Institute/Wellcome Trust Collaboration and former staff of the World Health Organization. Technical editing of the book has been completed by the Malaria Consortium, an international non-government organisation dedicated to control of malaria and supporting malaria programmes in many countries.

The editorial team at different stages of the book's development included: Kathy Attawell, Jane Edmondson, Jenny Hill, Sylvia Meek, Sunil Mehra, Julia Mortimer and Jayne Webster. James Tibenderana reviewed the complete draft. The authors are Bernard Brabin, Daniel Chandramohan, Christopher Curtis, Jane Edmondson, Mike English, Jenny Hill, Jo Lines, Sylvia Meek, David Robinson and Jayne Webster.

About the authors and editors

Kathy Attawell has worked in communications, previously with the international non-government organisation AHRTAG, and has extensive editing experience including a number of malaria publications. She has also worked on project management in public health and reproductive health in India and elsewhere.

Bernard Brabin is Professor of Tropical Paediatrics at the University of Liverpool, based at the School of Tropical Medicine. His research interests include maternal and child health and nutrition, perinatal and adolescent health, with a focus on developing countries. He has worked in Papua New Guinea, Kenya and Jamaica, and currently collaborates on community and hospital based studies in several African countries. He acts as a Technical Advisor to the WHO, European Commission and several research funding bodies. He holds an Honorary consultant appointment in Community Child Health at the Royal Liverpool Children's Hospital NHS Trust, Alder Hey. He was appointed in 1999 to the Foundation Chair of Tropical Child Health at the Academic Medical Centre, University of Amsterdam, which is held as a joint appointment with the University of Liverpool.

Daniel Chandramohan is a clinical epidemiologist based at the London School of Hygiene & Tropical Medicine. His main research interests include malaria, meningococcal meningitis and the methodology of measuring cause specific mortality. He has worked in malaria control programmes in Ethiopia and Zimbabwe, and currently he runs clinical trials in Ghana and Tanzania.

Chris Curtis has worked on malaria mosquito control based at the London School of Hygiene & Tropical Medicine since 1976, with field work especially in Tanzania. He has worked mainly on Insecticide-Treated Nets with some work on Indoor Residual Spraying and has supervised PhD students working on larval control. He has supervised masters students from many countries. He is Emeritus Professor of Medical Entomology.

Jane Edmondson's background is in management of health and health research in UK and developing countries. She spent two years in Uganda on a district health management strengthening project and then as a Management Adviser to the National Malaria Control Unit. At the time of writing Chapter 7, Jane was working for the Malaria Consortium at the London School of Hygiene & Tropical Medicine, providing consultancy support to African malaria control programmes and to the Roll Back Malaria Partnership. She now works as a Health Adviser for the UK Department for International Development in Pakistan.

Mike English is a Wellcome Trust Senior Research Fellow based at the Kenya Medical Research Institute (KEMRI) Centre for Geographic Medicine Research, Coast. He is a paediatrician in the Department of Paediatrics, University of Oxford and an Honorary Lecturer in the Department of Paediatrics, University of Nairobi. His main interests are the delivery of child and newborn health services in Kenya. By improving our understanding of the threats to survival in early infancy, his studies should result in a more informed approach to prevention and clinical care in the first vulnerable months of life.

Jenny Hill was Deputy Director of the the DFID-funded Malaria Consortium Resource Centre (1995–2003), based at the Liverpool School of Tropical Medicine (LSTM). She is now Research Project Manager in the Child and Reprodctive Health Group at LSTM and manages a Bill and Melinda Gates Foundation project to devise an integrated and prioritised global research strategy for malaria in pregnancy for the next five years, with the overall aim that optimal interventions will be developed and used in control efforts to reduce the adverse effects of malaria in pregnancy.

Jo Lines is a senior lecturer at the London School of Hygiene & Tropical Medicine and a member of the TARGETS communicable disease research programme consortium. His research has included environmental vector control, sampling methods, intervention trials, methods of treating and assessing insecticide-treated nets (ITNs) and implementation strategies for ITNs, including the role of the private sector and subsidised delivery systems. He has been a member of various WHO committees and working groups. He has worked closely with the Malaria Consortium, especially in the design and evaluation of malaria intervention programmes. He has worked in Tanzania, Ghana, The Gambia, Nigeria, Senegal, Kenya, Uganda, India, Venezuela, Thailand and Cambodia.

Sylvia Meek is the Technical Director of the Malaria Consortium. She previously worked with WHO in Solomon Islands, Namibia and Cambodia and with the World Food Programme and UNDP setting up and running vector-borne disease control programmes for refugees, and with UNDP in Equatorial Guinea. She was Director of the LSHTM and LSTM based Malaria Consortium Resource Centre. Her work includes technical advice especially on disease control policy, treatment policy, programme design, management and evaluation, consultancy management and technical leadership and strategy development of the Malaria Consortium.

Sunil Mehra is the Executive Director of the Malaria Consortium responsible for managing over 25 projects in Africa and Asia and is recognised for strategic planning and programme development in areas of maternal and child health, communicable diseases control and communications. He has worked in over 20 countries in East and South Asia, the Middle East and Africa.

Julia Mortimer was the Manager of the DFID Malaria Knowledge Programme from 1999 to 2004, based at the London School of Hygiene & Tropical Medicine. She is now Managing Editor of the Cochrane Collaboration's Heart Review Group.

David Robinson worked at the World Health Organization's Headquarters in the Division of Child Health and Development, then as a public health consultant. He played a leading role in development and implementation of the Integrated Management of Childhood Illness (IMCI) approach, and contributed to the sections on IMCI in this book.

James Tibenderana is the drug policy change specialist/epidemiologist for the Malaria Consortium Africa, prior to which he undertook doctoral research on management of severe malaria in Uganda and at the London School of Hygiene & Tropical Medicine. He coordinates the DFID Uganda-funded support to the drug policy change process in Uganda. This includes consensus building, training materials and guideline development, health worker training, drug availability in the private sector, use of rapid diagnostic tests and improving management of severe malaria. Previously, he has worked as a medical doctor at central and district levels in Uganda on communicable disease control.

Jayne Webster has a background in laboratory sciences and established a basic pathology laboratory in a remote area of Nepal. She is now a lecturer with the TARGETS Consortium at the London School of Hygiene & Tropical Medicine, and is currently focusing on monitoring and evaluation of delivery systems for public health interventions, particularly insecticide-treated nets.

We hope that this book will be a useful contribution to the work of front-line health professionals. We hope also that it will ensure health professionals have the basic information they need to take up the challenge of controlling malaria more effectively than ever before.

Introduction

Jenny Hill and Sylvia Meek

In this handbook we aim to provide basic information on malaria and its control for health professionals working in places where there are few published materials. The book provides essential information about malaria and practical steps for the main malaria control interventions. These are for people who carry out malaria control activities, people who need to plan such activities or who supervise others undertaking these activities. It is particularly designed for district health staff, but may be a useful reference book for health staff at other levels, students and teachers.

We have included some references for further reading: these can be found at the end of most chapters. In particular, anyone who needs a more detailed account of topics covered in this book is strongly recommended to look at *Essential Malariology* edited by Warrell and Gilles (fourth edition).

The world problem of malaria

For hundreds of years malaria has been one of the most important human diseases in the world. An eradication campaign in the 1950s and 1960s was effective in eliminating the disease from some parts of the world, mainly in parts of Europe and North America, and in reducing it in other places. Notwithstanding this success, *malaria still kills over a million people each year and causes between 300 and 500 million clinical cases.* Approximately 80% of the deaths and 90% of the clinical cases occur in sub-Saharan Africa, where young children and pregnant women are particularly at risk. Every year about a million children under five years of age die from malaria. Malaria also remains a major public health problem in Asia and parts of Latin America, where the disease affects people of all ages. Malaria disproportionately affects poor countries and communities, and hinders socio-economic progress of individuals, households and countries.

In spite of concerted efforts to control the disease, in many places the malaria situation is worsening. Malaria is increasing in many countries where it had been dramatically reduced (for example, India) or even eradicated (for example, parts of Eastern Europe). Now more than a third of the world's population live in malarious areas. Factors contributing to this worsening situation include increasing resistance to available drugs, changes in population immunity, population movements and climate change.

What can be done about malaria?

Malaria can be controlled. A number of methods are currently available for preventing or treating malaria. These methods include:

- elimination of the parasite through the identification and treatment of malaria cases or prevention of infection with drugs (chemoprophylaxis)
- reducing the mosquito vector population (with insecticides, biological or environmental methods)
- reducing the risk of being bitten by mosquitoes (using mosquito nets treated with insecticide or repellents).

Global and regional malaria control strategies

In 1992, at a Ministerial Conference convened by the World Health Organization (WHO), health ministers from all over the world endorsed a *Global Malaria Control Strategy*. It was based on an earlier strategy developed in the Africa Region, but used the basic principles of malaria control that apply throughout the world. How these principles are applied will depend on local variations in the disease and on the social, economic and institutional circumstances of individual countries and communities.

In 1998, the *Roll Back Malaria (RBM)* Partnership was formed. The partnership, founded by the World Health Organization, the United Nations Children's Fund, the United Nations Development Programme and the World Bank, includes governments, development agencies, civil society, professional associations, commercial organisations, research groups and the media.

RBM's goal is to halve the world's malaria burden by 2010.

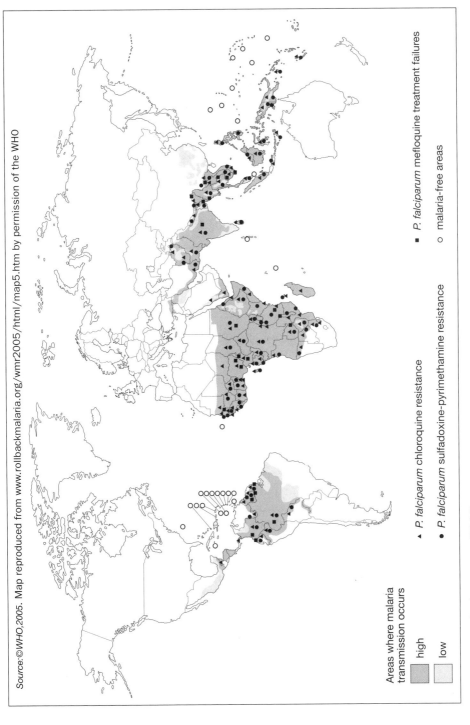

Source: ©WHO,2005. Map reproduced from www.rollbackmalaria.org/wmr2005/html/map5.htm by permission of the WHO

Areas where malaria
transmission occurs

high

low

▲ *P. falciparum* chloroquine resistance

● *P. falciparum* sulfadoxine-pyrimethamine resistance

■ *P. falciparum* mefloquine treatment failures

○ malaria-free areas

Malaria transmission areas, 2005

The six elements of Roll Back Malaria are:
- ▶ evidence-based decisions using surveillance and appropriate responses, as well as building community awareness
- ▶ rapid diagnosis and treatment
- ▶ better multi-pronged protection using insecticide-treated mosquito nets to control mosquitoes and making pregnancy safer
- ▶ focused research to develop new medicines, vaccines and insecticides and to help epidemiological and operational activities
- ▶ co-ordinated actions for strengthening existing health services and policies, and for providing technical support
- ▶ harmonised actions to build a dynamic global movement.

Integration with other parts of the health system

During the malaria eradication campaigns in the 1950s and 1960s, many malaria control activities focused solely on malaria, and did not consider other parts of the health services. Nowadays, we realise that we can only control malaria effectively if we make all parts of the general health services function well. We need to work with Ministry of Health policy makers and implementers, research institutions, in-service training programmes and information, education and communication (IEC) programmes to help people to protect themselves from malaria. We also need to consider nursing, technical and medical schools, drug distribution systems, health management information systems and health facilities. In addition, it is important to recognise that the public sector alone cannot control malaria and that involvement of the private sector is critical.

Within the context of integrated health systems, it is still important for a country with malaria to maintain specialist expertise in malaria control. Many countries have a malaria control unit, division or department within the Ministry of Health to run the National Malaria Control Programme (NMCP). Its responsibilities generally include co-ordination, planning, developing policies and guidelines, data analysis, and providing advice and training to other parts of the health service. Further malaria expertise, for instance on treatment guidelines, may be provided by a national advisory committee or special advisory groups.

Health sector reforms and decentralisation

A further change is happening in the organisation of many countries' health services. Decentralisation means that Ministries of Health give more responsibility for planning and managing health services to regional, district or sub-district levels, rather than making all decisions at central level. In some countries the districts have considerable responsibility for resources and the authority to decide how to use them. The decentralisation process may affect other parts of government services, so district administrators must make important choices on how to raise income and use their resources for different public needs, for example education, roads, agricultural development as well as health.

Decentralisation has some major advantages for malaria control. Malaria problems vary widely from place to place, so different responses are needed in different places. If local staff have the knowledge, skills and resources to tackle locally specific problems such as epidemics, the response will probably be quicker and more effective than if decisions are made at a higher level.

There are also risks in decentralisation. Many of the poorest countries have few resources for recruiting and training people in malaria control, so skills may be limited even at central level and very limited at district level. There may also be conflicting demands on limited resources, and the priorities of some district authorities may be determined by short-term and visible needs.

District staff now have greater responsibilities to analyse and understand their own situation, to respond to changes, to make informed decisions and to provide good quality, effective services as economically as possible. Districts urgently need skilled staff, who have the tools to carry out these responsibilities. Chapter 7 provides guidance for district level managers on planning and management.

Further reading

Warrell, D.A. and Gilles, H.M., Eds. *Essential Malariology*, Arnold, 2002, fourth edition

1 The Biology of Malaria

Sylvia Meek and Jenny Hill

This chapter discusses:

► the parasite that causes malaria, showing how the parasite moves from the mosquito to the human

► the mosquito that transmits malaria.

It describes:

► aspects of mosquito behaviour that are important in planning malaria control strategies.

It will be useful for primary health care workers, and also those who are interested in consolidating or extending their knowledge of malaria biology.

Introduction

Malaria is a disease caused by infection with a **parasite** (*Plasmodium*) which is transmitted from person to person through the bite of a female *Anopheles* mosquito. The mosquito picks up parasites from the blood of an infected person and injects them into the blood of another person, thereby transmitting the infection from person to person.

The parasite

The parasite that causes malaria is a single-celled organism or protozoon belonging to the genus *Plasmodium*. Within this genus there are almost 120 different **species** of *Plasmodium*, but only four species which infect humans. These are:

Plasmodium falciparum
Plasmodium malariae
Plasmodium ovale
Plasmodium vivax

6

Other species of malaria parasite infect a range of different animals.

The life cycle of the human malaria parasite has several stages. (See Figure 1.1 below; note that the **hypnozoite** stage occurs in *Plasmodium vivax* but not in *P. falciparum* – see page 8.) The sexual phase (**sporogony**) takes place in the mosquito where male and female parasites mate. The asexual phase (**schizogony**) occurs in the human, and has two stages:

1   **exo-erythrocytic schizogony** – multiplication of parasites in the liver, in the parenchyma **cells (hepatocytes)**
2   **erythrocytic schizogony** – parasite development in the blood-stream, in the red blood cells (**erythrocytes**)

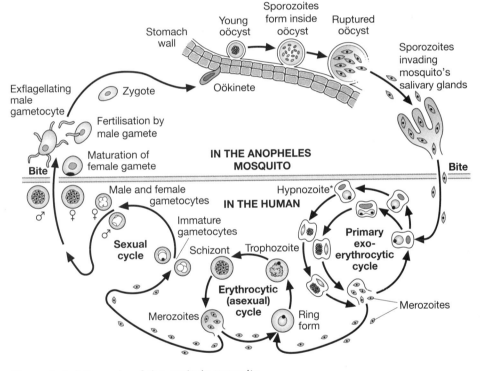

Figure 1.1: Life cycle of the malaria parasite

Note: Hypnozoites do not develop in P. falciparum or P. malariae.

Development of the parasite in the mosquito

The female *Anopheles* mosquito picks up malaria parasites when she sucks the blood of an infected person. Parasites found in human blood will be at different stages of development. Some infected people will only have asexual stage parasites: these will be digested and destroyed by the mosquito along with the blood she has sucked. Some people will also have parasites in their blood which are at the mature sexual stage. These are known as male and female **gametocytes** and they will develop inside the mosquito.

The developmental stages of the malaria parasite are as follows:

- The nucleus of the male gametocyte divides into eight nuclei, and each of these forms a long thread-like part called a **flagellum** (plural: flagella) or male gamete or **microgamete**.
- The flagella break out of the gametocyte, wave about for a few minutes, then separate. This process is called **exflagellation**, and can be seen in fresh blood with a microscope.
- The female gametocytes mature into female **gametes** or **macrogametes**.
- The male and female gametes fuse to form a zygote.
- Within 24 hours the zygote stretches into a moving oökinete which squeezes through the wall of the mosquito's stomach.
- The oökinete turns into a small ball-shaped oöcyst which attaches itself to the outside wall of the stomach. There can be up to several hundred oöcysts in one mosquito.
- Long thin **sporozoites** form inside the oöcysts, and burst out into the mosquito's body cavity, from where they go to the mosquito's salivary glands.

When the female mosquito bites a person, she injects saliva into the wound and may thus inject the malaria sporozoites at the same time.

Development of the parasite in the human

When the mosquito injects sporozoites into a person's blood, many are destroyed by the **host's** immune system, but the rest enter the liver's parenchyma cells within about half an hour.

The liver stage (exo-erythrocytic schizogony)

During the liver stage of the life cycle (sometimes called the tissue stage), the parasite undergoes two types of development:

- Pre-erythrocytic schizogony – this occurs as soon as the sporozoites reach the liver, where they develop immediately into pre-erythrocytic **schizonts**.
- Delayed exo-erythrocytic schizogony (only in *P. vivax* and probably *P. ovale*) – this occurs when some of the sporozoites reach the liver and turn into dormant single-celled hypnozoites. These do not multiply at first, but develop later into pre-erythrocytic schizonts. This causes a **relapse** in the disease, as these schizonts develop into blood stages. The length of delay

varies in different parasite strains, so in some countries *P. vivax* relapses quickly and in others it is much slower. Not all hypnozoites turn into schizonts at the same time, so there may be several relapses over a period of months (or even years), as new waves of hypnozoites begin to grow.

Development of the liver schizont takes six to sixteen days according to the species (see Table 1.1), and thousands of **merozoites** develop inside it. When the schizont is mature the liver cell splits, and the merozoites burst out into the liver tissue and then into the bloodstream.

The bloodstream stage (erythrocytic schizogony)

In the blood the merozoites enter the red blood cells (erythrocytes). This is the beginning of the erythrocytic stage.

The time between infection and when parasites first appear in the blood is called the pre-patent period. (This is different from the **incubation period** which is the time between infection and first appearance of symptoms of disease.) When a merozoite invades a red blood cell it becomes a **trophozoite** (*tropho-* means eating).

At first the trophozoite looks like a ring with a jewel, because it is shaped like a concave disk with the cytoplasm thicker at the edges than in the middle and the nucleus at the edge. (See Figure 1.1 above.) As it feeds on the contents of the red blood cell, it becomes globular and more irregular in shape.

After growing, the trophozoite divides asexually to form a schizont. This process is called erythrocytic schizogony. The trophozoite nucleus divides three to five times, and the cytoplasm divides with the nuclei. Each new nucleus with its attached **cytoplasm** becomes a rounded merozoite. The mature schizont contains between eight and 32 merozoites depending on how many times the nuclei divide. The red blood cell then bursts, and the merozoites are released into the bloodstream, where they invade new red blood cells and start developing into more schizonts.

This erythrocytic cycle of schizogony is repeated many times, so that more and more red blood cells become infected until either the person's immunity slows it down or drugs kill the parasites. Extensive damage to the red blood cells leads to anaemia and, if not treated, eventually to death.

The length of one cycle, from invasion of the red blood cell by a merozoite to invasion of another blood cell by the next generation of merozoites, differs in different species. It is 48 hours in *P. falciparum*, *P. ovale* and *P. vivax* and 72 hours in *P. malariae*.

Table 1.1: Features of the four species of human malaria parasite

Feature	Species			
	P. falciparum	P. malariae	P. ovale	P. vivax
Duration of sporogony in mosquito at 20°C (days)	22	35	?	16
Duration of sporogony in mosquito at 28°C (days)	9–10	14–16	12–14	8–10
Duration of pre-erythrocytic stage (days)	5.5–7	14–16	9	6–8
Pre-patent period (days)	9–10	15–16	10–14	11–13
Incubation period (days)	9–14	18–40 or longer	16–18 or longer	12–17 or up to 12 months
Duration of erythrocytic cycle (hours)	48	72	50	approx. 48
Number of merozoites in liver schizont (approx.)	30,000	15,000	15,000	10,000
Average number of parasites per µl (mm³) blood (**parasitaemia**)	20,000–500,000	6000	9000	20,000
Severity	Severe in non-immunes	Mild	Mild	Mild to severe
Relapses	No	No	Yes	Yes
Geographical distribution	Tropical and sub-tropical	Tropical and sub-tropical, patchy distribution	Tropical	Temperate regions and much of the tropics
Africa distribution	Most common species	West and East Africa	Quite common in West Africa	Less common especially in West Africa
Asia and Latin America distribution	Proportion varies	Guyana, India, Southeast Asia	Occasional in Southeast Asia	Proportion varies

Figures reproduced by permission of Edward Arnold (Publishers) Ltd

After the first few cycles of division, the parasites start to divide in time with each other, and this leads to the regular pattern of fever every few days (but see Chapter 3: Clinical and Parasitological Diagnosis of Malaria, as it is not completely regular). The *falciparum*, *ovale* and *vivax* malaria cycle is said to be three days, because the first fever is considered as day 1 and the second fever two days later is day 3. *P. malariae* has a four day pattern (fever on day 1 and day 4), and is called quartan malaria. (This is a little confusing as the three day pattern is actually every two days and the four day pattern every three days.)

Some merozoites do not divide, but develop instead into the sexual forms of the parasite called gametocytes. These are mainly produced after several rounds of blood schizogony as described above. The appearance of the different blood stages of the four species of human malaria parasites is described in Chapter 3: Clinical and Parasitological Diagnosis of Malaria.

The mosquito

Human malaria is normally only transmitted from person to person by certain members of the *Anopheles* genus (plural: genera) of mosquitoes. A small number of infections are also caused by blood transfusion from an infected donor or by congenital infection of babies whilst still in the womb. There are more than 400 species of *Anopheles* in the world, but only about 40 of these are important **vectors** (transmitters or carriers) of malaria. Only the female *Anopheles* mosquito transmits malaria to humans. Some *Anopheles* mosquitoes can also carry other human diseases, such as filariasis and some viruses. Two other genera of mosquitoes are significant in carrying other mosquito-borne diseases: *Aedes* is an important vector of the viral diseases yellow fever and dengue, and the *Culex* mosquito is an important vector of filariasis and Japanese encephalitis. It is useful to be able to tell the difference between these three types of mosquito if you are involved in **vector control**, so the main differences in each stage of the life cycle are shown in Fig. 1.2 on page 14.

The life cycle of the *Anopheles* mosquito

The mosquito has four main stages in its life: egg, **larva**, pupa and adult. It helps to understand the life cycle and natural history of the *Anopheles* mosquito, both to explain some aspects of the epidemiology of malaria and to find out the most effective ways to control the mosquito vector.

The egg stage

The female *Anopheles* mosquito lays batches of between 70 and 200 eggs in water every few days. They float on the surface of the water until hatching. The eggs are about 0.5 mm long. In tropical countries the eggs usually hatch two to three days after being laid, but take longer to hatch in cooler temperatures. They can survive for more than sixteen days on wet mud. Unlike *Aedes* eggs, they cannot survive drying out.

The larval stage

The egg hatches into a larva, which swims in the water and feeds. It needs to come to the surface to breathe air, but goes under water when disturbed. The larva has four size stages and sheds its skin (moults) between each stage. In tropical climates, the larval stage can be completed in just seven days, but in cooler temperatures it can take two to four weeks or may even last all winter.

The pupal stage

The larva develops into the pupa which is shaped like a comma. This stage lasts two to three days in tropical climates, longer in cooler climates. It does not feed, but must also come to the water surface to breathe air.

The adult stage

The adult mosquito then emerges from the pupa, often resting while its wings harden, then flies away. The adult mosquito body has three main parts: the head, thorax and **abdomen**. The head has large eyes, **antennae** and **palps**, as well as mouthparts known as the **proboscis**. The thorax has two wings and six legs. The antennae of the female mosquito have short hairs, whilst the antennae of the male have many long hairs, which look feathery. This is the easiest way to distinguish male and female mosquitoes.

The life span of the mosquito

The life span of the adult mosquito varies in different species. It is also affected by temperature, humidity, and the presence of hazards such as natural enemies and mosquito control measures. In humidity of less than 50% and a temperature greater than 35°C, the mosquito dies much sooner. In favourable conditions, female adults live on average ten to fourteen days, but some individuals will live much longer. Male mosquitoes live for a shorter time. The life span of the female is very important in the **transmission** of malaria, as it takes at least ten days for the malaria parasites in the mosquito to become infective to humans. Thus only the longer-lived mosquitoes will be able to transmit malaria.

Adult mosquitoes mate soon after emerging from the pupae. The female only needs to mate once, as she stores the male's sperm to fertilise each batch of eggs she produces. In most species she can only produce eggs after she takes a **blood meal** from a human or other animal. After she digests the blood and develops the eggs, she finds a suitable place to lay them. She then goes to look for another blood meal, and develops another batch of eggs. This cycle of feeding on blood and laying eggs is repeated for the rest of her life. It is called the **gonotrophic cycle**, and in tropical climates takes two to three days. Male mosquitoes do not feed on blood, but on nectar from flowers and other plant juices.

Identifying the main genera of mosquito

It is important to be able to identify the main genera of mosquito. There are three main ways to distinguish the adult of the anophelines (genus *Anopheles*) from culicines (which include genera *Culex* and *Aedes*).

1 The palps of male and female *Anopheles* are about the same length as the proboscis, and the male's palps are swollen at the ends. In the other genera the palps of the female are much shorter, while the male's palps are as long as the proboscis but never swollen.
2 Adult *Anopheles* normally rest at an angle (of approximately 45°) to the surface on which they stand. The other groups usually keep their body parallel to the surface (see Figure 1.2).
3 *Anopheles* mosquitoes' wings appear to have black and white spots, because the dark and pale scales on the wings are arranged in blocks. The other mosquitoes do not show these patterns.

The larvae of the *Anopheles* can also be easily distinguished from *Aedes* and *Culex*. They float flat at the surface of the water, whilst the other two hang down into the water with just their breathing tube at the surface.

Adult mosquito behaviour

There are several features of the behaviour of *Anopheles* mosquitoes which are important in understanding malaria epidemiology and in planning mosquito control. (It is also important to know the susceptibility of the mosquitoes to different insecticides when

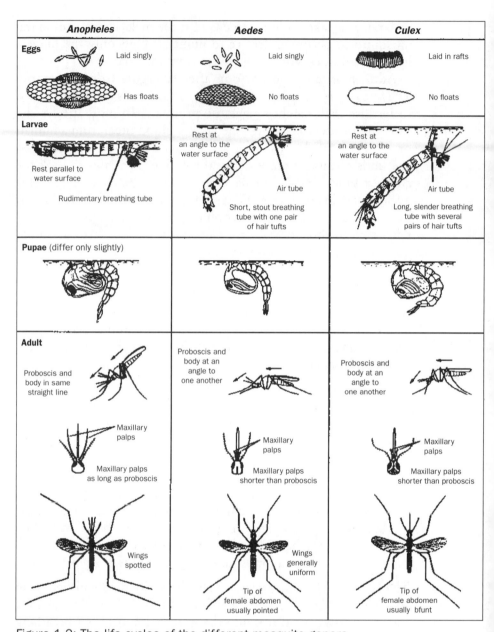

Figure 1.2: The life cycles of the different mosquito genera
(Source: *www.who.int/docstore/water_sanitation_health by permission of the WHO*)

planning vector control: for more on this see Chapter 5: The Prevention of Malaria).

Tables 1.2 and 1.3 on pages 18 and 19 show the important biological features of the major malaria vector species in different parts of the world.

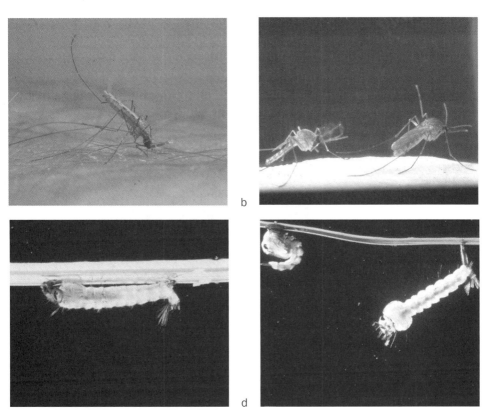

Figure 1.3: Mosquito types:
a *Anopheles* starting to feed
b *Culex* male and female
c *Anopheles* larva floating
d *Culex* pupa and larva hanging from the surface

Resting location

After taking a blood meal the female needs to find somewhere
to rest while she digests the blood and develops her eggs. Some
species remain inside the house, whilst others find resting places
outdoors. Indoor resting mosquitoes are more exposed to insecticide spray deposits in houses.

Feeding time

Almost all *Anopheles* take their blood meals at night, although a
few species occasionally bite during the day in dark places such as
thick forests. Each species has its own characteristic feeding time.
For instance, *A. farauti* in the Solomon Islands bites as soon as it

is dark, and mostly feeds in the early evening, whilst *A. gambiae* in Africa and *A. dirus* in Asia feed late at night. We might expect insecticide treated mosquito nets to work best where the vectors bite late at night, when most people will be in bed. However, this is not always the case: in the Solomon Islands, insecticide treated mosquito nets are said to work very well.

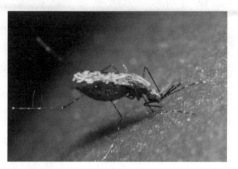

Figure 1.4: Beautiful *Anopheles gambiae* feeding

Feeding location

Some mosquitoes prefer feeding inside houses, others outside. Indoor feeding mosquitoes should be easier to control with insecticide treated nets or house spraying than those feeding outdoors.

Host preference

Different species of mosquitoes prefer different hosts. Clearly, the vectors of human malaria must feed on humans, but several species will feed partly on humans and partly on other animals such as pigs, dogs and cows. The species with a very strong preference for humans tend to be the most dangerous malaria vectors, as they are the most likely to pick up parasites and to pass them on.

Flight range

Most *Anopheles* mosquitoes do not fly more than two or three kilometres from where they began their life, so living more than this distance from **breeding sites** can reduce the risk of malaria. Occasionally mosquitoes travel further if carried by the wind – or even further if transported on vehicles such as ships and aeroplanes.

Breeding sites

Different species of *Anopheles* mosquitoes lay their eggs in different types of water bodies, but individual species tend to choose the same type. *Anopheles* mosquitoes do not normally lay their

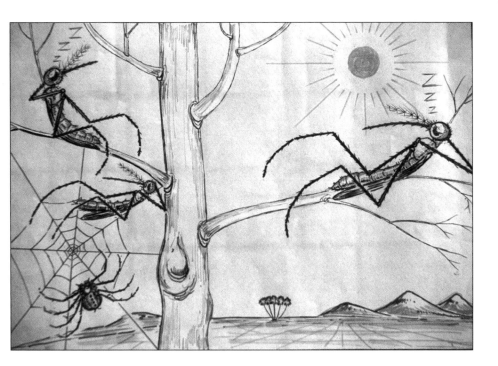

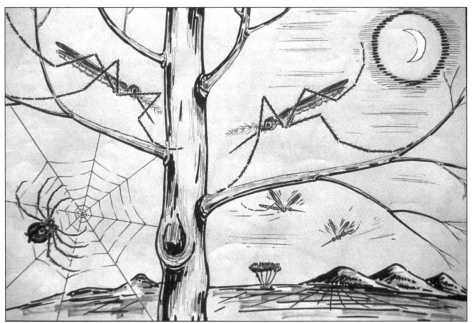

Figure 1.5: Visual aids used in health education talks.
    a Malaria mosquitoes rest during the day
    b They are active at night

(Source: Pathomasak Imvitya, United Nations Border Relief Operation, Thailand)

Table 1.2: Significant biological features of the major African malaria vectors

Anopheles species	Resting location	Feeding time/ location	Host preference	Breeding sites	Insecticide susceptibility
gambiae	Mainly in	Mainly late, indoors	Mainly human	Sunlit temporary pools, rice fields	Some resistance reports, recently to pyrethroids
arabiensis	In and out	Mainly late, in and out	Human and animals	Temporary pools, rice fields	
melas	Out and in	Mainly late, in and out	Animals and human	Salt water lagoons, mangrove swamps	
merus	Out and in	Mainly late, in and out	Mainly animals	Salt water lagoons, mangrove swamps	
funestus	Indoors	Mainly late, in	Mainly human	Semi-permanent and permanent water especially with vegetation, swamps, slow streams, ditch edges	

(Source: Mehra, S. *Partnerships for Change and Communication: Guidelines for Malaria Control*, 1995, reproduced by permission of the WHO)

eggs in polluted water. This is important when searching for the breeding sites of malaria vectors and deciding control measures (see Chapter 5).

The human

Clearly it is not just the biology and behaviour of the parasite and the mosquito which are important in the epidemiology and control of malaria. Human biology and behaviour are also important. For example, an individual's immunity level will determine how malaria affects them and how severely ill they become. A

Table 1.3: Significant biological features of the major and some minor malaria vectors of Cambodia, Laos, Myanmar, Thailand and Vietnam

Anopheles species	Resting location	Feeding time/ location	Host preference	Breeding sites	Insecticide susceptibility
dirus complex (7 sibling species; described as *A. balabacensis* in earlier literature	Mainly out	Mainly late (or 20– 02.00 hrs), out and in	Mainly human	Small shady pools mainly in forest and plantations, footprints, stream seepages, wheel ruts, gem pits, hollow logs, sometimes wells	Susceptible to DDT and others
minimus (at least 2 sibling spp)	Mainly out (previously in)	All night, mainly out (previously in)	Human and cows	Streams in forested foothills	Susceptible to DDT
maculatus complex (8spp.)	Mainly out	Peak 19– 20.00 or 21–24.00, mainly out	Mainly non- human	Sunlit streams. Sometimes ponds, tanks, riverbed pools	Susceptible to DDT and others
sundaicus (2 spp. suspected)	Out and in	All night, peak 20– 24.00 h, out and in	Human and domestic animals	Brackish or salt water near coast. Rockpools, river mouths	DDT resistance in Indonesia and Vietnam

(Source: *Vector Control in some Countries of Southeast Asia: Comparing the Vectors and the Strategies*, by S.R. Meek from Annals of Tropical Medicine and Parasitology, 1995, 89 135–147. Reproduced by permission of Maney Publishing. www.maney.co.uk/journals/atm)

person's behaviour also influences their risk of infection, for example the use of mosquito nets or coils, and influences their subsequent recovery if they do become infected, for example treatment-seeking behaviour. If people are given information and resources, and have the will to adapt their behaviour, much can be done to reduce the incidence of malaria. Good quality education strategies are thus an essential part of any malaria control programme.

Key points

> ▶ Malaria is a disease caused by infection with a parasite (*Plasmodium*) which is transmitted from person to person by the bite of a female *Anopheles* mosquito.
>
> ▶ The female *Anopheles* mosquito picks up the parasite that causes malaria when she sucks the blood of an infected person.
>
> ▶ There are four species of malaria parasite that infect humans, *Plasmodium falciparum, P. malariae, P. ovale* and *P. vivax.*
>
> ▶ The parasite develops in the mosquito into sporozoites which are infective to humans.
>
> ▶ When the mosquito bites a person, she injects saliva into the wound and at the same time may inject sporozoites contained in the saliva.
>
> ▶ These sporozoites may then be carried in the blood to the liver where they continue their development before invading red blood cells.
>
> ▶ Knowing the life cycle and natural history of the *Anopheles* mosquito helps in understanding malaria epidemiology and planning mosquito control.
>
> ▶ There are several features of the behaviour of mosquitoes which are important in understanding malaria epidemiology and in planning mosquito control. These include: resting location; feeding time; feeding location; host preference; flight range and breeding sites.
>
> ▶ Human biology and behaviour are also important in the epidemiology and control of malaria.

2 The Epidemiology of Malaria

Daniel Chandramohan

This chapter discusses:
► the practical use of epidemiological principles in thinking about malaria control.
It describes:
► the theoretical background for those who wish to gain a deeper understanding of epidemiological theories in relation to malaria control.
It will be useful for those working on national or regional malaria control programmes, and should also help district teams plan and evaluate their work.

Introduction

Epidemiology is the study of the distribution, frequency and determining factors of health problems and disease in human populations. The purpose of epidemiology is to obtain, interpret and use health information to promote health and reduce disease. Understanding the epidemiology of malaria is very important in deciding how best to use the available resources for appropriate malaria control activities.

One of the most important factors affecting the epidemiology of malaria is its pattern of transmission. This chapter begins with an overview of how different levels of malaria transmission are classified.

Classification of malaria transmission levels

Where does transmission of malaria occur?

Malaria occurs in many parts of Africa, Asia, Oceania and South America. *P. falciparum* is the most common species of parasite in areas of high endemicity (areas of high and regular malaria transmission) in Africa, Papua New Guinea and Haiti. *P. vivax* is the common species in Central America, North Africa, and southern and western Asia. Both species are present in South America and in the rest of Asia. *P. malariae* and *P. ovale* are found in areas where *P. falciparum* is common, but they cause much less malaria. However, in many parts of the world these patterns are changing. Levels of *P. falciparum* malaria are growing in areas where there is increasing **resistance** to commonly used anti-malarial drugs.

Identifying areas and levels of malaria transmission

Defining levels of malaria transmission at regional, country and **district** level allows the implementation of malaria control activities that are appropriate for the particular area. Where malaria is highly seasonal, it is important to identify peak transmission periods. This allows malaria control activities to be carried out in advance. Such activities include: retreatment of mosquito nets, rounds of indoor residual spraying (IRS), promotion of **prevention** techniques, and **health education** on the importance of prompt treatment-seeking. Those areas that are prone to epidemic malaria must be incorporated into an **early warning system** so that malaria control measures can be planned.

Classification of malarious areas

There are several terms used in describing the epidemiology and intensity of transmission of malaria. The term **endemicity** is used to describe the level of malaria transmission in an area. **Endemic** areas, where the **incidence** of malaria has been constant for many years (but may still have seasonal variations), contrast with **epidemic** areas, where increases in malaria are occasional and sharp. Traditionally, endemic areas are classified as hypoendemic, mesoendemic, hyperendemic and holoendemic.

- **Hypoendemicity** means that the level of transmission and the burden of malaria are low.
- **Mesoendemicity** is typically found in rural areas of subtropical zones where there are moderate levels of transmission.
- **Hyperendemicity** is found in areas with intense but **seasonal transmission** where immunity is inadequate to prevent the disease in all age groups.
- **Holoendemicity** is found in areas with intense year-round transmission where there is high immunity in all age groups except very young children. Areas with holoendemic malaria are often referred to as 'highly endemic'.

There are two ways of measuring the type of endemicity in an area.

Spleen rate is the prevalence of enlarged spleen among children aged 2–9 years

Parasite rate (PR), or parasite prevalence, is the percentage of people who have a positive blood slide test for malaria parasite (as measured through prevalence surveys).

Table 2.1: Classification criteria for endemicity of malaria

Level of endemicity	Spleen rate	Parasite rate (PR) in 2–9 year-old children
Hypoendemic area	<10% in 2–9 year-old children	Less than 10%
Mesoendemic area	<11–50% in 2–9 year-old children	11–50%
Hyperendemic area	<51–75% in 2–9 year-old children and >25% in adults	51–75%
Holoendemic area	>75% in 2–9 year-old children and low in adults	Over 75%

(Figures reproduced by permission of Edward Arnold (Publishers) Ltd)

Malarious areas are more broadly classified into **stable** and **unstable malaria**. The characteristics of these two epidemiological types of malaria are summarised in Table 2.2.

- In areas of stable transmission, malaria is endemic and often perennial (transmission throughout the year). Although there may be some degree of seasonal fluctuation, transmission remains high from year to year. Epidemics are unlikely.
- In areas of unstable transmission, malaria levels vary from year to year and epidemics are possible.

How would you classify malaria transmission in your district?
- ▶ Is malaria endemic or epidemic?
- ▶ If endemic, how would you define the level of endemicity?
- ▶ Is malaria transmission stable or unstable?

When are people at risk of malaria in your district?
- ▶ Is transmission perennial or seasonal?

Where are people at risk of malaria in your district?
- ▶ Does the endemicity of malaria vary in different areas?

Table 2.2: Characteristics of stable and unstable malaria

Characteristics	Stable malaria	Unstable malaria
Determinants of transmission		
Longevity of mosquito	long	short
Man-biting habit of mosquito	frequently feeds on human	infrequently feeds on human
Mosquito density required to maintain transmission	low (as low as 0.025 bites per person per night)	high (1–10 bites per person per night)
Suitability of climate	lasts for long periods	lasts for short periods
Indicators of the level and pattern of transmission		
Basic case reproduction rate	high	low
Incidence rate	usually high, particularly in younger children	usually low, similar in all age groups
Prevalence of immunity	high, though varies in different age groups	low
Seasonal changes in incidence	not very marked	marked
Epidemics	unlikely to occur except in migrants	likely when climate or other conditions are suitable
Potential to control transmission	very difficult to control	control is feasible

Assessment of malaria transmission levels

Measures of endemicity

Epidemiological measures used to assess the endemicity of malaria in an area (as well as any changes of this measure over time) include:

- incidence rate
- annual parasite index (API)
- prevalence.

Incidence rate

Incidence rate is the number of *new* cases of malaria per unit of population (for example, per 1000) per unit of time (for example, per year). If 2000 new cases are diagnosed in a year in a district with a population of 100,000 then the incidence rate is 20 per 1000 per year (2000/100,000).

However, it is often difficult to distinguish new infections from relapses and repeat infections. This makes it difficult to get a real measure of new cases, and so another measure – annual parasite index (API) – is sometimes used.

Annual parasite index (API)

API is the number of parasitologically confirmed **cases** of malaria per 1000 population per year. This means cases that are confirmed by blood slides (see Chapter 4: The Treatment of Malaria). API differs from incidence rate in that the parasitologically confirmed cases can be new, relapse or repeat infections.

Prevalence

Prevalence is the number of cases of malaria at a point in time per unit of population. For example, assume you test a **random sample** of 1000 people in one district for the presence of malaria parasites in their blood over a period of two weeks. If you find 100 of them to be positive for malaria, this means that the prevalence of parasitaemia (presence of parasites in the blood) in this population during the period of the survey was 10% (100/1000).

Both the incidence rate and the API may be calculated from routine health **data** that have been collected for other purposes. To calculate prevalence you will need to implement a **survey**. Note that the incidence rate and API calculated from routine health data only shows incidence among the population who use the health system. In many places, people often treat themselves at home and the incidence from health facility data can therefore underestimate the true extent of malaria.

Collecting data for assessing patterns of epidemiology

Data for assessing the epidemiology of malaria in your area may be collected through:

• **passive surveillance**
• **active surveillance**
• **sentinel surveillance**
• prevalence surveys.

There are also useful databases of information on malaria transmission patterns in Africa, available from Mapping Malaria Risk in Africa (MARA) – see below.

Malaria surveillance systems

Malaria **surveillance** is the ongoing and systematic collection, analysis, interpretation and dissemination of epidemiological and other data. It provides valuable information which may be used to answer questions on who is at risk, where they are at risk, and when they are at risk. The information is gathered in order to plan, monitor and evaluate malaria control programmes. It can also be used for early detection and control of **outbreaks** of malaria. Malaria surveillance systems mainly monitor the incidence of malaria in the population but can also include entomological measures (for example, mosquito density) and climatic variables (for example, rainfall). Choosing the most useful information to collect, with the resources you have available, is very important. In order to provide accurate data, you must have a clear **case definition** for malaria (see Box 2.1 below).

The surveillance system for malaria may be completely integrated with the general health information system for the country. Alternatively, each disease programme may have its own system, though they may still obtain some of their information from the general health information system.

Box 2.1: Malaria Case Definition

Any surveillance system should have a clear definition of a case of malaria. A typical case definition will be:

'a history of fever + presence of malaria parasites in a peripheral blood film'

Although the level of parasite density is useful to define a case of malaria more precisely in research settings, assessment of parasite density is generally not feasible in routine surveillance systems.

An incidence rate for clinical malaria that includes both cases confirmed by blood slide examination and unconfirmed cases may not be ideal to monitor the incidence of malaria. This is because the clinical diagnosis of malaria (diagnosis determined by assessment of symptoms) can vary depending on the knowledge and practice of the health workers, and by the prevalence of other fever-causing conditions.

However, in many developing countries, the majority of health units do not have the facilities to read blood slides and so the only information comes from clinical diagnoses. This can still be useful information, but needs to be interpreted carefully.

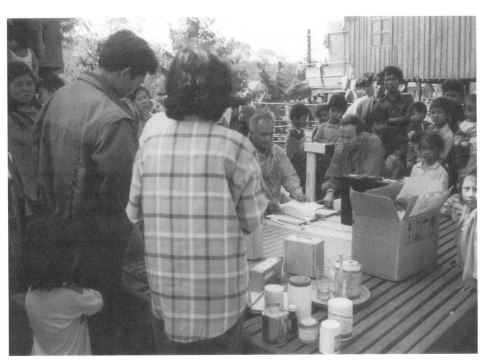

Figure 2.1: Malaria parasite survey, Cambodia

Passive surveillance

Passive surveillance is the secondary use of data that was collected for another purpose (such as the diagnosis and management of clinical episodes of malaria). The surveillance system may use the existing network of health facilities to obtain information on patients who present with fever or a history of fever. Sometimes records from village health workers are also included. Cases may or may not be confirmed by taking blood slides. However, in many countries private health practitioners do not participate in the passive surveillance system, so the incidence of malaria will be underestimated. Generally, passive surveillance systems cover the entire country.

Active surveillance

Alternatively, field workers may make weekly home visits and collect blood slides from anyone with fever or a history of fever. This type of active surveillance system is expensive, logistically difficult to organise, and may not be sustainable if you have limited resources. Although such systems were used to cover entire areas of operation during malaria eradication campaigns, they are probably not feasible or affordable for wide-scale use in a routine malaria control programme.

Sentinel surveillance

In a sentinel system, surveillance is restricted to a certain number of pre-selected areas. You can use either active or passive **case detection**. Ideally the areas you select should be reasonably representative of the various epidemiological and socio-economic situations found in the country. However, existing infrastructure, particularly transport and communication systems, may make some places more convenient than others. In epidemic-prone areas, sentinel surveillance systems may be important for early detection (see also Prevalence surveys, below).

Prevalence surveys

Parasite prevalence surveys use a **sample** of the population to provide a measure of the rate of parasitaemia in the population at the time of survey. When combined with clinical features, such as fever, they may also be used to estimate the rate of malaria disease in the population. However, it is important to remember that for the results to be generalised to the population from which the sample was taken, you must use randomisation techniques in the survey design. If you are planning a prevalence survey, you would be well-advised to seek the help of an epidemiologist. Prevalence surveys are expensive and time consuming.

MARA and MARA-Lite

For Africa, the Mapping Malaria Risk in Africa (MARA) website (*www.mara.org.za*) provides information on levels of malaria **risk** in different regions and sometimes districts. These data are also now available on a CD Rom called 'MARA-Lite'. The endemicity maps are not constructed using actual prevalence data, but use climate to forecast a likely model of endemicity. Historical prevalence data are, however, available on the website and on the CD Rom.

What factors determine the transmission of malaria?

The method by which malaria mosquitoes transfer malaria parasites between people is described in Chapter 1: The Biology of Malaria. The transmission of malaria depends on the following three elements:

- the host
- the agent
- the environment.

The host is the human being, and the agent is the malaria parasite. Mosquitoes also play host to the malaria parasite, but they are considered to be the agent of transmission, that is, the vector. The transmission of malaria is determined by the interactions among the host, the agent and the vector. The physical, biological and socio-economic aspects of the environment, in turn, influence these.

Host (human) factors

Important host factors that influence the risk and severity of malaria infection include:

- natural resistance
- **acquired immunity**
- age
- pregnancy
- beliefs and practices
- migration.

These are discussed below.

Natural resistance

Some individuals have inherited conditions that give them a degree of resistance to malaria infection. For instance, people with red blood cells that lack a protein called 'Duffy blood-group antigen' have marked resistance to *P. vivax* infection. Similarly, the presence of haemoglobin S in an individual's blood (which causes sickle cell anaemia) can reduce the severity of *P. falciparum* infections.

Acquired immunity

Individuals who are exposed to repeated infections of malaria, over a period of several years, become semi-immune. This means that although they are still at risk of infection when bitten by an infected mosquito, they either do not have symptoms (are **asymptomatic**), or their symptoms are not severe. Unless the individual is continually re-infected, full immunity to malaria will not develop and the semi-immunity that has developed will fade.

Semi-immunity develops in several stages. Firstly, the **signs and symptoms** of malaria become less severe for a given **parasite density**. In other words, as a person acquires immunity, he or she needs to have more parasites in the blood to suffer the same degree of malaria disease. Next, there is a gradual reduction in the density of parasites (gametocyte and asexual stages) in the blood. This then leads to a reduction in the prevalence of the parasite in adults and older children when compared to children under five (before they acquire semi-immunity). In highly endemic areas, older children and adults will therefore often have very low level asymptomatic parasitaemia.

Age

Generally, where malaria is common, children will be more susceptible to infection than adults because they will not yet have acquired immunity. In highly endemic areas, such as much of sub-Saharan Africa, malaria is a disease of children – 80% of one-year-old children in these areas may be parasitaemic. In areas of low endemicity such as parts of Asia, where most people are non-immune, all age groups are equally prone to infection.

Pregnancy

In endemic areas, women who are semi-immune become more susceptible to malaria during pregnancy. This is especially true if it is their first pregnancy. For those women who have no immunity to malaria, the risk of severe **outcomes** of malaria is increased. (See Chapter 6: Malaria in Pregnancy.)

Beliefs and practices

People's beliefs about diseases (causes, prevention, cure) will influence their practices, and this can have an important effect on the transmission of malaria. For example, many people recognise that mosquitoes are a nuisance, but do not know that they can cause malaria. This will affect their attitude towards preventing mosquito bites by using mosquito nets, fly curtains, mosquito repellents or protective clothing. Similarly, sleeping habits, treatment-seeking behaviour, attitudes toward malaria control measures such as residual insecticide spraying and insecticide treated mosquito nets can all affect the transmission of malaria.

Migration

Human migration is often associated with malaria transmission. People with no immunity may move from a non-malarious area into a malarious area. Conversely, carriers of malaria parasites from a malarious area may take the parasite into areas with little or no malaria and with no immunity in the population. Either of these events can change the pattern of transmission in a given area.

> Who is at risk of malaria in your district?
> ▶ Which age groups?
> ▶ Are pregnant women likely to be semi-immune?
> ▶ What beliefs and practices are likely to affect risk of infection
>   and severity of disease?

Agent factors

The malaria parasite

As explained in Chapter 1, four species of malaria parasite can cause infection in human beings (*P. falciparum, P. vivax, P. malaria* and *P. ovale*). Within each of these four species, there are several strains with different epidemiological characteristics. Different strains will have different antigenic properties, so being immune to one strain may not make a person immune to others. Because new strains appear regularly, it is difficult for people to acquire total immunity to malaria parasites.

The vector

There are over 60 species of *Anopheles* mosquitoes that can transmit malaria. However, there are rarely more than four different species in a particular geographic region. Different species of mosquito may vary in their breeding sites, feeding and resting habits, and longevity (life span). For example, *A. gambiae* (an important vector in sub-Saharan Africa) breeds in rain pools, while *A. culicifacies* (a common vector in Asia) breeds in freshwater streams.

Several key mosquito factors determine the capacity of mosquitoes to transmit malaria which, in turn, determines the level of transmission of malaria:

- density
- **man-biting habit**
- longevity.

Measurement of these factors is performed by specialised entomologists and is not routinely conducted at district level, as it often expensive and time consuming. It is, however, useful to consider these factors when thinking how different species of vector may affect the levels of malaria transmission in your district.

Density

This is the number of vectors present in a place in relation to the human population. For example, if, on average, 400 female *anopheline* mosquitoes were found daily in 10 houses where 40 people live then the mosquito density will be 10/person (400/40).

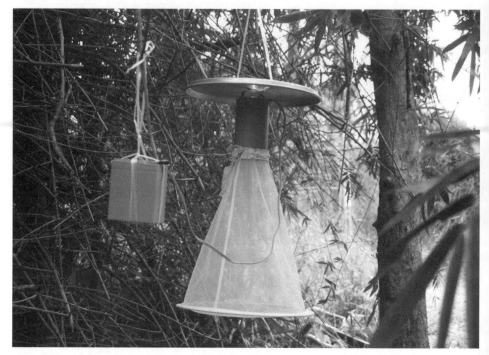

Figure 2.2: Using a CDC light trap to collect adult mosquitoes to assess the effectiveness of vector control on the Thai-Cambodian border

The man-biting habit

This measurement is a combination of how often the female mosquito takes a blood meal and the choice of host (see Box 2.2 below). The frequency of feeding depends on the species of mosquito and on the temperature. The choice of host is determined by the species and also by the availability of alternative hosts for feeding. The man-biting habit is measured as the number of times per day that the mosquito feeds on humans. The more times a mosquito bites a human per day, the greater the chance that it will deliver an infected bite and therefore transmit malaria.

The example opposite shows that *A. gambiae* has a higher man-biting habit than *A. culicifacies*.

Box 2.2: Man-biting habit

> *A. gambiae* typically feeds once in two days ($\frac{1}{2}$ feeds per day) at optimum temperatures and usually only on human beings (100%). Thus the man-biting habit is:
>
> $\frac{1}{2} \times \frac{100}{100} = 0.5$ feeds per human per day
>
> *A. culicifacies* feeds once in three days (or $\frac{1}{3}$ feed per day) and only a proportion (10%) of them feed on human beings. Thus the man-biting habit is:
>
> $\frac{1}{3} \times \frac{10}{100} = 0.03$ feeds per human per day

Longevity

The incubation period of the parasite in the mosquito (the **extrinsic** cycle) is the interval between the day it picks up gametocytes from an infective human being and the first day on which sporozoites are present in its salivary glands, ready for transmission.

The incubation period will rarely be less than ten days. Thus, only mosquitoes that become infected and then survive through the incubation period (at least ten days) can transmit the infection. Generally, the probability of dying, per day, for a mosquito does not depend on age. It depends heavily on environmental conditions and varies greatly between species of mosquito.

Environmental factors

The transmission of malaria is affected by *temperature* and *relative humidity*.

- When the temperature is below 16°C, malaria parasites cannot develop in the mosquito.
- Within a temperature range of 19 to 33°C, the incubation period in the mosquito (extrinsic cycle) of *P. falciparum* varies from ten to 30 days.
- Within a temperature range of 15 to 32°C, the incubation period for *P. vivax* varies from eight to 30 days.
- A high relative humidity lengthens the life span of the mosquito, allowing it more time to deliver more bites and thus transmit infection to more people.

- When the mean temperature ranges between 20–30°C and the relative humidity is more than 60%, development of the malaria parasite in the mosquito and its transmission will be at its maximum.

An increase in surface water from *rainfall* is generally associated with an increase in mosquito density, and hence in malaria transmission.

- Rainfall increases the number of breeding sites.
- There is higher relative humidity after rainfall, lengthening the mosquito's life span.

During a drought, however, rivers that are normally too fast-flowing for certain species of *Anopheles* to breed may become strings of pools more suitable for breeding. Excessive rainfall may, in some areas, lead to a reduction in transmission if small streams become rapid torrents that wash away the aquatic stages of the mosquito.

Socio-economic factors

Factors such as type of housing, sanitation, education and occupation can have a significant effect on the transmission of malaria. They can alter the level and patterns of contact between mosquitoes and human beings.

Epidemics of malaria

An epidemic of malaria means that the incidence rate, during a particular time period, exceeds the normal rate in the area by a given (excessive) amount. Epidemics occur in areas of unstable malaria where most of the conditions for intense malaria transmission exist, but where one or more essential factors are usually missing. If the missing factor appears, the environment needed for transmission will be complete, and an epidemic or outbreak will result. In such areas, malaria incidence will normally be low, or there will be no transmission, so the population will have little immunity to malaria.

Where and when do epidemics occur?

Any one or a combination of the following conditions can lead to an epidemic:

1 An increase in the number of susceptible people in a malaria endemic area, for example migration of non-immune individuals, such as displaced people, into an endemic area

Box 2.3: Epidemic or outbreak?

The terms 'epidemic' and 'outbreak' are often used as if they mean the same thing. However, these may be distinguished as:

▶ epidemics involve large numbers of people over a wide geographical area
▶ outbreaks involve a relatively small number of people within a smaller area.

Differences between epidemics and outbreaks can also be defined by how much the incidence of malaria has increased.

2 An increase in the number of people carrying parasites in an area of low endemicity, for example migration of people carrying malaria parasites from a highly endemic area into a low endemic area

3 An increase in **vectorial capacity**, for example changes in rainfall and temperature that increase the longevity, frequency of feeding or density of mosquitoes

4 The introduction of more efficient mosquito vectors into a malaria endemic area

5 An increase in breeding sites through large-scale development projects, such as the construction of dams

6 The discontinuation of vector control techniques, especially indoor residual spraying, or the breakdown of control programmes during emergency situations.

Epidemics of malaria are generally associated with greatly increased mortality. Thus early detection – supported by a prompt and effective response – is vital.

Early warning systems

The purpose of an early warning system is to predict the timing and likely severity of an epidemic. Methods used for predicting epidemics include those that detect the risk of increased malaria transmission, and those that detect an increase in the **vulnerability** of the population or of particular groups within the population. The first priority when considering an early warning system for malaria epidemics is to establish whether the district is, in fact, prone to epidemics. If the district is epidemic prone, it is important to define the reasons for this and the factors known to have sparked epidemics in the past. For example, if certain climatic factors, such as early rains, pose an epidemic risk, then the monitoring of rainfall would be a key element of an early warning system.

Transmission risk indicators (climatic monitoring)

Climatic changes can often be used as transmission risk indicators. They may predict an increase in malaria transmission a few months before it occurs.

Seasonal climate forecasts can be used to predict those climatic changes at regional and national levels that may affect malaria transmission. During El Niño years, some regions experience drought, while some regions may have above average rainfall. Similarly, some regions are warmer and others are cooler than average. Fluctuations in temperature and rainfall during El Niño years have corresponded with variations in the incidence of malaria and with epidemics in certain regions, such as northwestern India and East Africa.

In order to make the most of this information, there needs to be good collaboration and communication between meteorological services and malaria control programmes. Meteorological data are available to health services in many countries through national weather centres. These measure and record rainfall, temperature and sometimes humidity from a number of weather stations. You can use such local, regional and national level monitoring of weekly rainfall levels to predict the potential for an epidemic in some areas. Generally, above average rainfall is likely to increase mosquito density. However, in certain areas, below average rainfall may increase mosquito density and longevity, depending upon the species of mosquito and their breeding preferences. Predicting early rain in some areas will enable the preparatory phase of control to get underway. Further confirmation of the rainfall pattern would then allow time to mobilise vector control activities.

Vulnerability indicators

For an epidemic to occur there must be a large number of susceptible (vulnerable) people who are likely to become clinically ill when they are exposed to infection. The number of people who will be vulnerable to severe malaria depends upon the levels of immunity and therefore upon malaria endemicity (see pages 34–35). In areas of high endemicity, pregnant women and children under five are vulnerable. In areas of highly seasonal malaria and low endemicity, all age groups are vulnerable. Vulnerability indicators will not help you to determine the likely timing of an epidemic, but they will help you predict the severity of the impact of an epidemic.

You should also consider movement of human populations as a potential cause of an epidemic, when the movement is either from or to a malarious area. This could be movement during complex emergencies and natural disasters – of people as **refugees** or as **internally displaced persons** (IDPs). You can assess the potential risks by looking at the malaria transmission levels in the areas of origin and destination, and also in the areas through which the populations pass en route. For Africa, the Mapping Malaria Risk in Africa (MARA) website (*www.mara.org.za*) and the MARA-Lite CD Rom provide information on levels of risk of different regions, and sometimes districts. Although they are not highly accurate, these resources can give an indication of likely levels of protective immunity in different populations.

Health facility data indicators

Health facility data can be used to confirm the presence of an epidemic and to help in predicting its magnitude. You should consider any unusual increase in the number of malaria cases, both clinical and confirmed, as detected through routine surveillance (see page 26) as a potential epidemic and investigate it. To detect an increase in incidence in malaria cases, you need to know the expected incidence of malaria in the given geographic area over a particular period of time. However, even when data on the incidence of malaria over several years are available, it can be difficult to estimate the expected incidence. This is because over the course of a year, most areas will have a natural variation in the intensity of transmission. A five-year rolling average of the monthly incidence of malaria may be useful as a baseline rate. The sensitivity of health facility data within an early warning system can be improved by receiving information from peripheral services, via emergency channels. This could include events such as abnormal increases in fever cases, or the risk of running out of anti-malarials.

Investigation and control of epidemics

Verifying the occurrence of an epidemic

The first stage in determining whether an epidemic is actually occurring is to assess whether the number of malaria slide positive cases is higher than you would expect at the given time of the year. You should increase the use of blood slide examination from fever cases through passive surveillance and, if necessary, start active surveillance in the affected locality. The use of rapid diagnostic tests is recommended in the verification of epidemics (see Chapter 3, page 74) as a small team of people can accurately screen many patients in one day.

Organising control measures

Once the epidemic has been verified, a rapid response should be put into action, and will need good co-ordination of people able to help. Appropriate control measures include:

- health education campaigns
- mass treatment in some circumstances, where feasible and necessary – this should be considered where there is high mortality, and where at least 80% of fever cases at health facilities or at home are shown to be malaria
- measures to control adult mosquitoes and to reduce contact between humans and mosquitoes – indoor residual spraying, in particular, may be an effective response to eliminate adult mosquitoes, provided it is started early enough
- intermittent preventive treatment for pregnant women.

Investigating the factors contributing to the epidemic

You will need to carry out a rigorous assessment of the potential factors that could have led to the epidemic. These include migration, climatic changes, failure of control programmes and drug resistance. You will also need to evaluate the effectiveness of the early warning and surveillance systems.

Reporting on the epidemiology and control of the epidemic

Lessons learned from any epidemic will be useful for the prevention and control of future epidemics. A systematic record of the events of any epidemic should be compiled, analysed and disseminated. Your report should include:

- **morbidity** and **mortality rates** in children and adults
- a graphic presentation of the distribution of cases and deaths by week (**epidemic curve**)
- an analysis of the **effectiveness** of the early warning and surveillance systems
- a description of the control measures carried out
- an analysis of potential factors contributing to the epidemic
- recommendations for the prevention and control of future epidemics.

Key points

> ▶ It is important to define malaria transmission levels (endemicity) at district, regional and national level so that appropriate control activities may be implemented.
>
> ▶ At the district level it is important to determine whether malaria
> – is endemic or epidemic
> – if endemic: at what level?
> – transmission is stable or unstable
> – transmission is perennial or seasonal
> – transmission varies in different areas of the district.
>
> ▶ The epidemiology of malaria in your area may be assessed through passive surveillance; active surveillance; sentinel surveillance; and/or through prevalence surveys.
>
> ▶ The transmission of malaria depends upon the host, the agent and the environment, and the interactions among all these elements.
>
> ▶ Early detection of epidemics, together with a prompt and effective response, is important to prevent an increase in mortality.
>
> ▶ If the district is epidemic prone, it is important to define the reasons for this and the factors that have previously sparked epidemics. These risk factors should then form the basis of an early warning system.

Further reading

1 Snow, R., Gilles, H.M. (2002) 'The epidemiology of malaria' in Warrell, D.A. and Gilles, H.M., Eds. *Essential Malariology*, Arnold, 2002, fourth edition, pp 85–106
2 Bouma, M., van-der Kaay, H. 'The El Niño Southern Oscillation and the historic malaria epidemics on the Indian subcontinent and Sri Lanka: an early warning system for future epidemics?' *Tropical Medicine and International Health*, 1996, 1: 86–96
3 Hay S., Renshaw M., Ochola S., Noor A., Snow R. 'Performance of forecasting, warning and detection of malaria epidemics in the highlands of western Kenya' *Trends in Parasitology*, 2003, 19:394–399

3 Clinical and Parasitological Diagnosis of Malaria

Mike English and Jayne Webster

This chapter describes:

► the range of diagnostic methods

► the assessment of the signs of severe disease

► how to take a medical history

► how to conduct a physical examination

► how to make a diagnosis

► how to assess the severity of malaria

► how to use different parasitological diagnostic methods.

It will be useful for health workers in primary health care facilities who are responsible for diagnosis, including those who treat patients and need to make a clinical diagnosis or request laboratory tests, and those who work in the laboratory. It can also be used by managers who are developing and running health facility systems.

Introduction

Malaria control strategies emphasise the need for early diagnosis of malaria cases in order to reduce morbidity and mortality. Patients with *P. falciparum* malaria who do not receive prompt and effective treatment may progress to severe malaria within a few hours to days.

Diagnosis of malaria ideally means a clinical judgement, based on symptoms and signs, supported by a parasitological diagnosis to test for the presence of parasites in the blood. (Parasitological diagnosis is often described as laboratory diagnosis, but some tests, for example rapid diagnostic tests, do not require a laboratory.) Clinical judgement should include assessment of whether the malaria is uncomplicated (mild) or severe, and what complications are present. In some parts of the world, it is also important to know which type of malaria parasite is present. In practice, in many malaria endemic areas of the world, the majority of people do not have **access** to health units with laboratory facilities and so most treatment is based on a clinical diagnosis alone. If you carry out the clinical diagnosis incorrectly (either diagnosing malaria when it is something else, or the other way round), the results can be extremely serious. It can mean delayed recovery, the increased risk of serious complications and death – and it can contribute to the development of drug resistance. It is therefore important that clinical diagnosis is carried out as accurately as possible. Where laboratory facilities are available, these can obviously greatly improve the accuracy of the diagnosis. However, clinical judgement is still vital, since the presence of malaria parasites in the blood does not always mean that the patient is suffering from malaria. (Many people in highly malaria endemic areas will have malaria parasites in their blood without being ill due to malaria; see Chapter 2: The Epidemiology of Malaria.) Ideally, diagnosis of malaria should be based on:

- a complete history of the condition
- a physical examination
- laboratory investigations.

As the choice of first-line malaria treatment in many countries changes to artemisinin-based combination therapy (ACT), the importance of increasing use of parasitological diagnosis where possible has been recognised to avoid treating patients with no parasites. This is partly because ACTs are much more costly than most older treatments and also to reduce the risk of more resistance development. Some patients treated without malaria may subsequently be infected when the drug levels in their blood are too low to kill all parasites. In highly endemic areas of Africa, treatment of children under five based on clinical diagnosis is appropriate to minimise the risk of missing cases, but parasitological diagnosis may be more widely recommended for older children and adults.

The most appropriate approach to diagnosis will depend on where you are (and hence the likelihood that your patient could be infected with malaria); the likely type of malaria, and the patient's risk of developing serious complications. The use of clinical and laboratory diagnosis is therefore discussed at different levels of endemicity, and at the various levels of health facility:

- In areas where people rarely experience malaria, they do not develop immunity (see Chapter 2). Infections in such non-immune people may lead to severe disease, which may affect most organs of the body. This is generally the case in South and Southeast Asia and other areas of the world where malaria is present but not highly endemic.

• In areas where people are constantly infected with malaria, they develop semi-immunity (see Chapter 2). Those who are semi-immune to malaria may develop mild malaria, but are protected from developing severe malaria. Populations in many parts of Africa and Papua New Guinea develop such semi-immunity.

Increasing movement of populations, and possibly some climate changes, are causing malaria to occur in areas where it was previously almost unknown. Malaria should now be considered as a possible cause of symptoms in many areas, and enquiries about exposure (for example, questions about travel) should therefore be made. The minimum time after arriving in a malarious country, when symptoms can be attributed to malaria (incubation period) is about seven to nine days (see Chapter 1: The Biology of Malaria). The maximum period after exposure to infection risk when the patient may still have malaria can be as long as twelve months for *P. vivax*. Malaria should also be considered even where a patient has a history of **anti-malarial prophylaxis** use, as visitors from non-endemic areas may be at much higher risk of developing severe disease.

Box 3.1: Those most at risk of developing severe malaria

Health workers should be aware of those most at risk of developing severe malaria. These include:

▶ children in areas of high endemicity, especially those aged six months to five years
▶ people of all ages in areas of low endemicity; travellers from areas where there is little or no malaria
▶ those returning to highly endemic areas after several years' absence
▶ pregnant women, especially those in their first pregnancy
▶ immunosuppressed people.

Clinical diagnosis

Clinical diagnosis involves using the patient's symptoms and signs to decide what illness or combination of conditions he or she has. The process of diagnosis includes:

- assessing quickly for signs of severe disease
- taking a medical history
- conducting a physical examination
- making a **differential diagnosis**
- ordering laboratory tests (if available)
- making a provisional diagnosis
- deciding a prognosis.

Assessing for signs of severe disease

It is important that you make a quick assessment for signs of severe disease, so that treatment may be started immediately, and the patient referred where necessary. Clinical features such as witnessed **convulsions, prostration, coma** and respiratory distress (all described below) indicate that the patient needs urgent clinical assessment and treatment.

- Convulsions are most common in **febrile** children. They may be obvious, or they may also present in subtle ways. Important signs of convulsions include rapid, jerky eye movements (intermittent **nystagmus**); salivation; and minor twitching of a finger, toe or corner of the mouth.
- You need to test actively for prostration: it presents as an inability to drink or breastfeed (if less than one-year old) and an inability to sit unsupported (if one year or above).
- Coma is an inability to fix or follow objects with the eyes in children under eight months of age, and the inability to localise a painful stimulus if aged eight months or over.
- Respiratory distress is deep breathing and/or in-drawing of the lower chest wall.

Where any of the signs listed above is present, you need to assess the patient immediately, start treatment and make a referral if necessary (depending upon the level of your facility). (See also Chapter 4: The Treatment of Malaria.)

Taking a medical history

Patients usually present for consultation with health workers because they have symptoms of disease. Your first task as a health worker is to document these symptoms, and obtain further information that will affect decisions on diagnosis. The purpose of taking a history is to look for clues to assist diagnosis.

Box 3.2: Symptoms and signs

Symptoms
Symptoms are indications of a disease or disorder that can be noticed by the patient, such as fever.

Signs
Signs are indications of a medical disorder that are elicited or measured by a medical practitioner, such as body temperature.

Ask the patient or parent questions on:
- *Symptoms* – their timing and duration: ask about fever, chills and **rigors** (shaking of the body), headache, joint weakness or tiredness; in children ask also about common childhood symptoms such as cough or difficulty breathing, diarrhoea, ear pain or measles within the last three months.
- *Geographical history* – where they live and where they have travelled recently.
- *Drugs taken already* – anti-malarial and other drugs taken before and during this illness.
- *Previous illnesses and treatment* – especially recent febrile illness, and sickle cell anaemia and diabetes, both of which may contribute to the clinical picture.
- *Previous blood transfusions* – because hepatitis may resemble malaria, or malaria may itself be transmitted by transfusion.
- *Pregnancy* – it is important to check whether the patient is pregnant, in order to assess risk and determine appropriate treatment.
- *Other illnesses in the family* – which may suggest an alternative diagnosis.

Conducting a physical examination

Basic observations

The first part of a physical examination is basic observations; do these for all patients. Basic examinations include:

- weight
- state of nutrition, for example underweight or wasted
- temperature – either measured in the axilla, mouth or rectum
- colour of mucous membranes and white part of the eyes
- dehydration (eyes sunken, mouth dry, fast pulse, inelastic skin)
- pulse rate
- blood pressure (if needed)
- respiration rate and type of respiration
- **oedema**
- **splenomegaly** (i.e. an enlarged spleen).

Follow basic observation by an examination of the part of the body which the symptoms and signs suggest may be diseased. If the disease you think the patient has is one that affects more than one part of the body, or you are not certain of the diagnosis, conduct a full body examination. Assess the patient quickly but thoroughly.

Systemic examination for malaria

Central nervous system

Assess the level of consciousness of the patient. If he or she is in coma, use a coma scale based on whether the patient is able to open his or her eyes, move or speak in response to either painful stimuli or verbal commands (see Table 3.3).

Respiratory system

- Count respiratory rate, look for fast or deep laboured breathing.
- Look for chest in-drawing, especially in children.
- Listen to the chest for rales (**crepitations**) or any added sounds.

Cardiovascular

- Take pulse, including the rate and volume.
- Check for cold extremities.
- Check capillary refill time.
- Take blood pressure.
- Listen for heart sounds.

Abdomen

- Feel the spleen and liver for enlargement.
- Loin tenderness may be indicative of **pyelonephritis**.

Common clinical features of uncomplicated and severe malaria

The presentation of both uncomplicated and severe malaria is variable and non-specific. Patients may also have more than one underlying disease. There are, however, several clinical features of both uncomplicated and severe malaria (see Table 3.1) which are common in both adults and children (unless specified), and in those who are semi-immune and non-immune. Note though that none of these is specific to malaria alone.

Clinical features of uncomplicated malaria

High-grade fever is the main feature of uncomplicated malaria. However, patients may also complain of headache, muscle pains, joint pains and/or weakness, chills and rigors. Some people may just feel 'unwell'. In young children, common complaints are loss of appetite, abdominal pain and vomiting. Uncomplicated malaria is generally classified as the presence of the above clinical features, singly or in combination, with or without laboratory confirmation. Where there is a national definition, this should be adopted.

Clinical features of severe malaria

Severe malaria means *P. falciparum* malaria that is sufficiently serious to be an immediate threat to life. As with uncomplicated malaria, the diagnosis of severe malaria is based on clinical features and confirmed by laboratory findings. However, for severe malaria, while laboratory testing should not delay the onset of treatment, it is essential that you have a laboratory diagnosis. It is important to remember, however, that a negative blood film does not necessarily exclude a diagnosis of severe malaria. In severe malaria, it is possible that the parasites will not be detectable by microscopy because they have been sequestered in the deep tissues of the brain. Diagnose a patient as having severe malaria if there are asexual forms of *P. falciparum* on a blood film, and if a history and physical examination indicate that they have any of the following:

- change of behaviour – confusion, drowsiness, agitation, hallucinations or psychosis
- altered consciousness or coma – which may be moderate or profound, and gradual or sudden in onset
- convulsions – with signs including movement of the hands and face, biting of the tongue and incontinence
- **hypoglycaemia** (low blood sugar) – which may manifest as altered behaviour, loss of consciousness, convulsions, sweating and cold, clammy skin
- acidosis – deep (not necessarily rapid) breathing is a good indication of acidosis, but not entirely dependable because other factors may influence the breathing pattern
- difficulty in breathing – can be influenced by the effect of malaria on the brain, by **acidaemia**, by high fever, **pulmonary oedema** or respiratory distress syndrome, which is indistinguishable from pulmonary oedema but occurs in the absence of fluid overload
- **oliguria** or acute renal failure – which is detected by monitoring urine output
- severe **anaemia** (**haematocrit** less than 20%, Hb less than 6g/dl) – can only be properly diagnosed by measuring haematocrit or **haemoglobin** level, although signs suggesting severe anaemia include severe **pallor** of mucosae, especially the tongue
- circulatory collapse or shock – which is indicated by low blood pressure, a feeble pulse and impaired perfusion with cold, clammy skin and peripheral **cyanosis**
- **haemoglobinuria** – identified where the urine is dark and tests positively for blood (haemoglobin), but contains no red blood cells on microscopy
- jaundice – which is best detected on the sclerae of the eyes
- a bleeding tendency – there may be spontaneous bleeding from the gums or in the skin, tested through monitoring bleeding time
- prostration – extreme weakness where the patient cannot walk or sit up without assistance.

It is important to consider other possible diagnoses, because a patient may have any one or any combination of these complications. Most patients will also have fever, but not all will. Absence of fever does not exclude a diagnosis of severe malaria. Patterns of fever are not very helpful in making a diagnosis, because *P. falciparum* malaria in particular can cause a very irregular fever pattern.

Table 3.1: Clinical symptoms seen in uncomplicated and severe malaria

	Uncomplicated	Severe
General	fever rigors (adults) muscle aches backache vomiting lethargy dehydration	fever rigors pallor – pale **palmar** creases and mucosal membranes in the eye and mouth severe lethargy and prostration dehydration: – reduced skin turgor – poor urine output poor capillary refill clinical acidosis frank haemoglobinuria jaundice
Neurological	headache	coma or impaired consciousness (see text and Table 3.3) fits neck stiffness (mild) arching of the back gaze abnormalities (divergent gaze) tooth grinding (**bruxism**) extensor posturing and rigidity retinal **haemorrhages**
Cardiovascular	tachycardia	**tachycardia** mild **hypotension** ± mild **postural hypotension** poor peripheral perfusion: – cold hands and feet – capillary refill > 2 seconds very poor peripheral perfusion: – weak peripheral pulses – capillary refill > 5 seconds shock
Respiratory	in children: cough and **tachypnoea**	in children: chest in-drawing, grunting and nasal flaring crackles cyanosis
Abdomen	**hepatomegaly** splenomegaly	hepatomegaly splenomegaly

Duration of symptoms

Severe disease is a progression from mild disease. If you treat mild disease promptly and effectively, it will not progress through to severe disease. In adults, severe malaria generally develops after several days of milder symptoms, but in children, severe malaria can develop very quickly with death occurring within 24 to 48 hours of the first signs of illness. Duration of symptoms is, therefore, rarely useful in distinguishing mild from severe malaria, especially in children.

Making a differential diagnosis

A differential diagnosis is a statement of the possible causes of the complaint. Malaria must be considered in the differential diagnosis of any acute febrile illness in a patient.

Malaria shares many symptoms with several other infectious illnesses listed in Box 3.3 below. These diseases will not all be familiar to all health professionals, as they occur in different parts of the world. The overlap in symptoms makes clinical diagnosis of malaria difficult. The relative prevalence of both malaria and these other infectious diseases will vary by area, and so differential

Box 3.3: Infectious diseases that share clinical features with malaria

Any febrile illness that may cause a febrile convulsion
Infectious mononucleosis (glandular fever)
Influenza
Leptospirosis
Meningitis
Pneumonia or viral lower respiratory tract infection
Acute psychoses
The relapsing fevers
Scrub typhus
Septicaemia
Trypanosomiasis
Typhoid (enteric fever)
Viral encephalitides (e.g. Japanese B encephalitis, rabies)
The prodromal phase of viral exanthema in children (e.g. roseola)
Viral haemorrhagic fevers (e.g. dengue)
Viral hepatitis

diagnosis will also vary. Taking a careful history is important, as it will help to provide a firm basis for differentiation between malaria and any other diseases that may be responsible for the symptoms seen. In clinical diagnosis, the factors that may influence what differential diagnoses are considered, and what symptoms and signs are most common, include:

- the background level of malaria in the **community**
- whether or not other infectious diseases that may be confused with malaria also occur in the community
- age
- pregnancy
- previous self-treatment for malaria.

These factors are all included in the section on Taking a medical history (see page 44).

In general, in a low risk area and in the absence of alternative explanation for a patient's fever, you can base a clinical diagnosis of uncomplicated malaria on his or her exposure to malaria, plus a history of fever with no features of severe disease. In children and pregnant women from high transmission areas, you should regard the presence of palmar pallor as malaria, unless there is an obvious alternative cause of the pallor. In older children and adults, you should base clinical diagnosis on fever. However, in many parts of Africa, incidence of malaria may be low in adults and older children, so look for other causes of the fever.

Signs suggesting an alternative diagnosis

It is important that you carry out a physical examination to identify any other possible causes of the illness, and to assess the severity of the malaria and any of its complications. Before considering malaria as the sole cause of clinical problems, make sure that you exclude other possible causes of symptoms and signs. This is particularly important with meningitis, pneumonia or septicaemia, which present a similar clinical picture.

In all patients, signs suggesting an alternative diagnosis include:

- rash – which is rare in malaria and may indicate measles, typhoid or other illness
- neck stiffness – which may be a sign of meningitis
- **sepsis** – in any limb or organ
- enlarged lymph nodes – which may indicate tuberculosis, AIDS related infections or other illness.

In children, signs suggesting an alternative diagnosis include:

- inflammation behind eardrums – which may indicate acute or chronic **otitis media**
- inflamed pharynx – could indicate tonsillitis or diphtheria
- bulging **fontanelle** – suggests meningitis in small children
- **koplik spots** of prodromal measles on **buccal mucous** membranes
- shallow, rapid breathing with nasal flare – may indicate acute respiratory infection or pneumonia.

One approach widely adopted to ensure that the major causes of childhood mortality are adequately treated, and that multiple illnesses are not missed, is **Integrated Management of Childhood Illness**. This is introduced in Box 3.4 below.

Box 3.4: Classification of illness in Integrated Management of Childhood Illness (IMCI)

IMCI employs guidelines and training materials designed to give first-level facility health workers skills in managing the conditions that most commonly cause mortality in children in developing countries (pneumonia, diarrhoea, malaria, measles, malnutrition). (The various components of IMCI are described more fully in Chapter 4: Treatment of Malaria.) IMCI uses a clinical algorithm to classify children based on the treatment they need. IMCI is not a diagnosis in the clinical or pathological sense; it is a classification which depends upon the sign and symptom complexes defined by the algorithm.

Depending upon classification of the illness (or more often illnesses), the result is an urgent referral to a higher-level health provider (possibly with some essential treatment immediately), specific medical treatment and advice, or simple advice on home management.

The current IMCI algorithm proposes the assessment, classification and treatment of malaria without the need for microscopy. The need to consider changing the approach to include parasitological diagnosis is being discussed, as the introduction of more costly anti-malarial drugs necessitates more emphasis on rational use of these drugs.

Distinguishing malaria species

P. vivax, P. ovale and *P. malariae* very rarely cause life-threatening disease, although there may be complications. Frequent episodes of malaria (particularly *vivax* malaria) in young children may reduce growth. It is difficult to distinguish these forms of uncomplicated malaria from *P. falciparum* uncomplicated malaria through clinical diagnosis alone. Laboratory diagnosis is necessary to identify the species of infecting malaria parasite and can be useful in deciding what treatment to use. It can also be useful in assessing the possibility of progression to severe disease. However, even in a laboratory, it can be difficult to differentiate malaria species, and **mixed infections** of *P. vivax*, *P. ovale* and *P. malariae* malaria with *P. falciparum* malaria are common in some areas.

Ordering laboratory tests

As clinical diagnosis alone is unreliable, it is important that appropriate laboratory tests are conducted where there are facilities and trained people to do this. You need to have a blood film prepared to demonstrate the presence and species of asexual parasites. It is important, however, to remember that:

- obtaining a blood film result must not delay starting treatment
- occasionally blood films can be negative even though a patient has severe malaria. If clinical features strongly suggest severe malaria, treatment should be started even if blood films are negative.

In settings where laboratory investigation is not possible, you should start patients who have symptoms of severe malaria on anti-malaria treatment as soon as possible, despite the poor reliability of clinical diagnosis.

Making a provisional diagnosis

The provisional diagnosis is the condition that you think the patient really has. This should be decided after the differential diagnosis has assessed all the conditions that could cause the symptoms and signs seen in the patient.

Deciding a prognosis

The risk of mortality depends on several factors, including degree of abnormality of symptoms and signs, age, immunity, and access to effective treatment. Features which indicate that a patient is at increased risk of dying include being unable to swallow tablets, evidence of vital organ dysfunction and a high **parasite count**. The complications encountered in severe malaria are described in the following section.

Assessing the severity of malaria

It is important to remember that the clinical features of severe malaria differ with age. As explained above, in areas where transmission of malaria is high and stable, severe malaria is mainly a disease of young children (i.e. below five years of age). The semi-immunity acquired by older children and adults protects them against severe outcomes of malaria. In areas of low transmission, severe malaria may occur in all age groups. WHO's identification of the defining features of severe malaria in adults and children focuses mainly on these two categories. The presence of any one of these features, as described in Table 3.2, is a cause for concern. (See also Box 3.5 on page 54.)

Table 3.2: Differences in the clinical features of severe malaria in adults and in children*

Clinical feature	Children	Adults
History of cough	common	uncommon
Convulsions	very common	common
Duration of illness	1–2 days	5–7 days
Resolution of coma	1–2 days	2–4 days
Neurological sequelae	>10%	<5%
Jaundice	uncommon	common
Pretreatment hypoglycaemia	common	uncommon
Pulmonary oedema	rare	uncommon
Renal failure	not usually	occurs
CSF opening pressure	usually raised	usually normal
Respiratory distress (acidosis)	common	sometimes
Bleeding/clotting disturbances	rare	up to 10%
Abnormality of brain stem reflexes (e.g. oculovestibular, oculocervical)	more common	rare

(*Derived from studies in Southeast Asian adults and children, and African children)
(Figures reproduced from *Management of Severe Malaria: a practical handbook*, WHO, 2000, second edition by permission of WHO)

Box 3.5: Defining features of severe malaria: Definitions and comments

Cerebral malaria is defined as unrousable coma not attributable to any other cause in a patient with *P. falciparum* malaria and can be recognised by the inability to localise a painful stimulus.

Repeated generalised convulsions are so common in children with malaria that they may not be a useful sign of severe disease.

Severe anaemia is defined as a haematocrit less than 15% or haemoglobin less than 5 g/dl which is normocytic in nature and associated with a parasitaemia of more than 10,000/µl. This may be too strict a definition in clinical practice, particularly in African children.

Renal failure is defined as a urine output of less than 400 ml in 24 hours in an adult or less than 0.5 ml/kg/hr in a child which fails to improve after adequate rehydration and is associated with a serum creatinine more than 265 µmol/l (more than 3.0 mg/dl).

Pulmonary oedema is difficult to diagnose reliably without a chest x-ray. When it is severe, it may show itself as frothy pink secretions in the mouth, but more commonly it causes a rise in respiratory rate, more effort needed to breathe, the development of cyanosis if oxygen is not given, and crackles can be heard in the lungs. In cases of fluid overload, the jugular venous pressure (or central venous pressure if measured) is high.

Hypoglycaemia is defined as a whole blood glucose concentration less than 2.2 mmol/l (less than 40 mg/dl). Clinically this may be difficult to diagnose, but suspect this in any patient (particularly children) with other features of severe malaria or any patient with impaired consciousness.

Shock is defined as a systolic blood pressure less than 50 mmHg in children aged 1–5 or less than 70 mmHg in older children or adults associated with clinical signs of poor perfusion (see Table 3.1).

Acidosis is defined as an arterial pH less than 7.25 or a plasma bicarbonate less than 15 mmol/l. This laboratory definition is of only limited value since blood gas analysis is often not available. However, at least in African children, it may be possible to diagnose a moderate to severe metabolic acidosis using clinical signs alone.

It is important that obvious *haemoglobinuria* (black, red or smoky urine) resulting from acute malaria infection is distinguished from that resulting from treatment with anti-malarial drugs, which is known to cause haemolysis in people with red cell defects such as G-6-PD deficiency.

Spontaneous bleeding usually occurs from the gums or nose and may be associated with skin petechiae (round, flat, dark red spots caused by bleeding into the skin or beneath mucous membrane) and/or sub-conjunctival haemorrhage. In such cases, laboratory tests of coagulation may be grossly abnormal (with evidence of disseminated intra-vascular coagulation, DIC). Spontaneous gastro-intestinal haemorrhage may also occur and be life-threatening. Thrombocytopenia (low platelets) is very common, but need not be associated with bleeding or other coagulation problems.

Clinical features of severe *P. falciparum* malaria

Neurological features

The term 'cerebral malaria' is frequently used to describe severe malarial disease. However, a number of different definitions of the term have been used in the past, because many patients with severe malaria have some neurological impairment (see Table 3.3) without being comatose. The term should therefore be used carefully to avoid confusion.

Coma

Coma is defined as 'the inability to react appropriately to a painful stimulus (usually pressure applied to the **sternum** with a knuckle) by attempting to remove the stimulus'. This is often referred to as an inability to 'localise' a painful stimulus. It is important for a clinician to distinguish between a *deliberate* attempt to remove the stimulus and the reflex movement of the arms towards the midline in response to pain, which is sometimes seen in patients with coma.

This is the simplest definition of coma, and is the one recommended by WHO for the diagnosis of cerebral malaria. Assessment of the coma score is based on the patient's ability to move and speak in response to commands and painful stimuli. You can do this by using the Glasgow Coma Scale (GCS) for adults and older children (see Table 3.3). For children aged nine months to five years, use the Blantyre Coma Scale (BCS), which is a modification of the

GCS (see Table 3.3). Measurement of coma in younger infants is more difficult. In infants who cannot yet speak, assessment should be made on the cry, the response to pain and the ability to watch the mother's face.

Table 3.3: Coma scales

	Glasgow coma scale			Blantyre coma scale	
	Adults	Score		Children	Score
Best motor response (to a painful stimulus where necessary, either to the sternum or to a limb)	obeys command	6		localises	2
	localises	5		withdraws limb from pain	1
	withdraws limb from pain	4		absent or other response	0
	abnormal flexion of limbs	3			
	extension of limbs	3			
	no response	1			
Best verbal response (to a question or, where appropriate, to a painful stimulus)	orientated	5		appropriate cry	2
	confused conversation	4		inappropriate cry	1
	inappropriate words	3		absent cry	0
	incomprehensible sounds	2			
	no response	1			
Eye opening/ visual response	spontaneous	4		directed (i.e. able to focus gaze)	1
	to speech	3			
	to pain	2		not directed (eyes may be open or closed)	0
	no response	1			
Total scored	maximum	15		maximum	5
	minimum	3		minimum	0

To obtain the coma scores, work out the score for each section and add the three figures to give a total score.

Remember the following when making a diagnosis of coma:

- Wait at least half an hour after the end of a convulsion.
- Do not diagnose immediately after the administration of anti-convulsant drugs – in other words, a repeat examination may be required to see if the patient has regained consciousness.
- In patients who have had very prolonged convulsions or received very large doses of anti-convulsants, particularly intramuscular diazepam (see Chapter 4), wait an hour or more before deciding that failure to localise indicates a malaria-induced coma.

Convulsions

Generalised convulsions in an adult who has no prior history of a seizure disorder are an indication of severe malaria. Convulsions are, however, less useful in defining severe malaria in non-immune children aged six months to five years – they may just have simple febrile convulsions. Prolonged (more than 15 minutes), focal or multiple convulsions might be better indicators of severe malaria in this group of children.

In 'semi-immune' children, convulsions, even when multiple, are extremely common in clinical malaria. Although this means that they are not particularly useful in defining severe disease, convulsions are still important. There is evidence that very prolonged convulsions (more than 30 minutes) – which are often referred to as 'status epilepticus' – are associated with neurological problems such as hemiplegia and cortical blindness that persist after recovery from acute malaria. Also, in some children, the electrical activity in the brain associated with convulsions may persist for hours. Although this causes only minor clinical abnormalities (for example, nystagmus, twitching of the lips or fingers alone, or irregular respiration) it can be entirely responsible for the 'coma'. Therefore, treating these subtle convulsions can sometimes result in the rapid resolution of 'coma'.

Severe anaemia

The usual definition of severe anaemia in malaria is:

*'a **normocytic** anaemia with haematocrit of less than 15% or haemoglobin less than 5 g/dl in the presence of parasitaemia more than 10,000/µl'.*

However, while this definition is useful in 'non-immune' adults or children, on its own it is a poor indicator of life-threatening malaria in children from highly endemic areas. In these children, you also need to look for signs of respiratory distress before considering severe anaemia as a sign of severe malaria.

Because iron deficiency is very common in this group, you should consider as severe malaria:

• severe anaemia (normocytic or microcytic), plus
• any evidence of *P. falciparum* malaria on laboratory testing (including the presence of malaria pigment alone), plus
• associated respiratory distress.

Renal failure and haemoglobinuria

Renal failure is one of the most common and important complications of severe malaria in adults. This is particularly true in Southeast Asia, where it also occurs in children. Urine which is black, dark red or smoky is a sign of frank haemoglobinuria. Occasionally, this haemoglobinuria may be the presenting feature in a patient who has no other signs of severe malaria, and such cases often progress to acute renal failure.

Although complete renal failure is very rarely observed in children from highly endemic areas, renal impairment and mild haemoglobinuria or haematuria (detected on urine dipstick) are more common than previously thought.

The most important aspect of assessment of renal dysfunction is ensuring that the patient is not dehydrated, as dehydration can cause poor urine output and a rise in creatinine. Look for simple clinical signs (reduced skin turgor, acidotic breathing, slow capillary refilling, sunken eyes) to estimate the degree of dehydration; the same signs can be used as for diarrhoea/gastroenteritis guidelines, and these are particularly useful in children.

Where facilities exist, you can use central venous pressure monitoring as a tool for deciding on fluid replacement therapy in adults.

Pulmonary oedema, circulatory collapse and shock

Pulmonary oedema is a very serious complication of *P. falciparum* malaria in adults, but is very rare in children from highly endemic areas. It occurs most often in three situations:

• as an isolated problem, sometimes associated with hyperparasitaemia
• in patients who have developed renal failure and are subsequently given too much fluid
• as part of a syndrome of multi-organ dysfunction or failure.

In the last group, patients may have renal failure, severe jaundice secondary to liver impairment, and cerebral symptoms. In such cases, pulmonary oedema may develop without any evidence of fluid overload.

Circulatory failure or shock can occur, together with multi-organ failure or before it develops. It is sometimes caused by another problem, particularly septicaemia. Circulatory failure rarely develops suddenly, so examine patients early for signs of poor perfusion and start treatment early.

Metabolic acidosis and respiratory distress

In adults, acidosis may occur together with renal failure and/or circulatory failure. Metabolic acidosis is an important feature of severe malaria, particularly in children, where it is most commonly associated with poor circulation and/or severe anaemia. As well as the clinical signs of poor circulation and anaemia (see Table 3.1), these children often have a characteristic form of breathing which is a common sign of respiratory distress (see Box 3.6).

Jaundice

In non-immune adults, jaundice is a relatively common finding and may reflect both liver dysfunction and **haemolysis**. Clinical signs of liver failure never indicate malaria alone.

In semi-immune children, jaundice is uncommon and is usually mild, and is never found as the only feature of severe malaria. Its importance is, therefore, not clear, but it does not require specific treatment.

Classifying severe disease in children

A simple approach to classifying severe disease in children who have been exposed to *P. falciparum* malaria from birth uses two major life-threatening complications:

- cerebral malaria
- severe anaemia (Hb less than 5 g/dl or PCV less than 15%).

Younger children tend to suffer from severe anaemia and older children from cerebral malaria, although either complication can happen at any age. These diseases are also affected by geographical factors. The age by which clinical immunity develops, and the specific pattern of disease in areas of constant exposure to *P. falciparum* malaria, are influenced by the intensity of malaria transmission. Severe anaemia in young children predominates in areas where transmission is high, while cerebral malaria is more common in areas where transmission is lower.

Although this simple classification of the clinical pattern of severe *P. falciparum* malaria in children in endemic areas is useful to epidemiologists, it is less helpful to clinicians in making decisions about treatment. However, severe malaria in 'semi-immune' children can be defined based on simple clinical bedside tests. These tests (see Box 3.6) are likely to be particularly useful in hospitals or **health centres** with very limited facilities where it is not possible to use the more complex criteria in Box 3.5 (page 54). Box 3.6 presents some of the features of severe disease that can be identified without sophisticated facilities.

Box 3.6: Other features of severe disease which can be identified where diagnostic facilities are limited: description and comment

Respiratory distress*
Principally applied to children, in whom it has been shown to be a very useful indicator of life-threatening disease when observed either as an isolated abnormality, or when associated with severe anaemia or neurological features of severe malaria. Experts have different views on the clinical signs that are most useful in diagnosing respiratory distress but the following are frequently used:

▶ nasal or alar flaring (flaring of the nostrils when breathing in)
▶ in-drawing/retractions/recession of the chest wall when breathing in (best observed at the lower margin of the chest wall)
▶ grunting (a grunting noise made when breathing out)
▶ deep or acidotic breathing (a regular pattern of breathing in which the chest expands markedly when breathing – like someone who has just been running fast).

Of these signs (which often occur together) deep or acidotic breathing is probably the most important, as it identifies children with metabolic acidosis who may require specific treatment (see Chapter 4).

Although the respiratory rate is frequently high when someone is suffering respiratory distress, the rate of breathing is not a particularly important feature.

Prostration*
This describes the state of a child or an adult who is conscious, but so lethargic or weak that they cannot sit up or drink without assistance. These patients can localise a painful stimulus, can understand and obey simple commands, are oriented and can make appropriate visual responses. In a young child, the key

to this diagnosis may be the ability to fix and follow an object (usually the mother or clinician) with the eyes. In children who are too young to be able to sit reliably (less than eight months) you can also regard inability to breastfeed as a useful alternative guide.

Neurological impairment
Some patients are able to localise a painful stimulus, but in other ways are clearly not in a normal state of consciousness. Such patients may be confused and/or unusually agitated, unusually sleepy or unable to respond appropriately to questions or commands. These patients might be described as neurologically impaired rather than in coma. In children, this term has been suggested for those with a Blantyre Coma Scale (BCS) score 3 or 4.

Hyperparasitaemia
The definition of hyperparasitaemia may vary with location. Thus parasitaemia involving more than 5% of peripheral red blood cells might be regarded as hyperparasitaemia in adults or children who have no immunity to malaria, whereas a parasitaemia more than 20% of peripheral red cells is often the definition of parasitaemia in African children living in highly endemic areas. Even with such apparently high parasitaemia in such children, however, there may only be a slightly increased risk of death than with lower parasitaemia. In other words, hyperparasitaemia is not always a good definition of severe malaria.

* Look for these features to define severe malaria in African children.

Case studies

1 *Sanjay returns from the farm and is sick*
Sanjay is 25 years old and went to see his local doctor complaining of *fever, headache, backache* and *feeling sick,* although he was not vomiting and had no diarrhoea. He had *recently returned* to the town from his farm, which was 40 miles away near the river. He usually spent several months of the year there and *had previously been treated for* vivax *malaria.* The doctor's clinic was very busy and in a quick examination, the only thing he could find was that Sanjay had a *red throat* and a slight *fever of 38°C.* The doctor prescribed some antibiotics for a throat infection and sent Sanjay home.

The following day Sanjay *was brought back to the clinic* by his brother because he felt *worse*. He *was able to talk* but *felt too weak to walk to the doctor's clinic*. He still had a *severe headache*, had felt very cold during the night and *could not stop shivering*. The doctor examined Sanjay more thoroughly and found, in addition to the red throat, that he could feel both the *liver and spleen*.

What do you think is wrong with Sanjay? Would you have managed this case differently?

Comment   Sanjay presented with very common symptoms – a fever and a red throat – which made the doctor think this was a throat infection. (Since most throat infections are caused by viruses, the antibiotics were probably unnecessary.) However, the doctor failed to note where Sanjay had recently been living and, since there was no malaria in the town, he had not considered malaria likely. The next day Sanjay was clearly worse, and had probably had a rigor. The enlarged liver and spleen may have been present the day before, but the doctor had not examined his abdomen.

By the second day, Sanjay had many of the signs of malaria. Since he had recently been living in a malarious area and had previously contracted the disease there, a malaria diagnosis should have been considered. If possible, an urgent sample should have been sent to a laboratory, and treatment for malaria given. Based on Sanjay's symptoms and signs alone it is impossible to tell if he has *vivax* malaria again or the potentially more serious *falciparum* malaria. His weakness raises concerns that he might develop severe malaria.

2   Ibrahim has a puffy face and swollen ankles

Ibrahim is six years old and living in an area where malaria is very common. He had been ill with malaria several times before. On this occasion, he developed a *fever* and his father gave him some *malaria tablets* which he had bought from a shop. The next day Ibrahim still had a fever, so his mother took him to the hospital where they examined his blood. The report from the laboratory showed a *few malaria parasites*, so he was given more anti-malarial treatment. He seemed to *get better*, but about a week later his mother noticed that he had a *puffy face and swollen ankles*.

What do you think was wrong with Ibrahim and what would you have done?

Comment   In areas where the disease is common, people often treat malaria at home. This can sometimes make it very difficult to detect malaria parasites and distinguish species in laboratory tests, which may be negative even if malaria is the problem. Ibrahim was infected with *P. malariae* and, although this was successfully treated, he developed one of the rare complications of this infection – nephrotic syndrome – which can be fatal. Sadly, there is little specific treatment to prevent this complication – it is a form of allergic response to the parasite. It is also important to remember that a few people have severe allergic reactions to some anti-malarial drugs, particularly drugs with a sulphonamide component.

3 Thien is unable to stand up or understand what is going on

Thien arrived at the health centre with another man who worked with him for *the logging company*. This man said that Thien had been unwell *for two days* with a *fever and generalised aches and pains*. He had sat with the other workers briefly the night before, but had not eaten anything. He had then gone to bed early, taking some medicine for fevers, which someone had given to him. In the morning they had found him in his bed *unable to stand up* and apparently *not able to understand* what they were saying.

The medical assistant examined Thien and found that he could open his eyes when his name was called, but that he could not tell them where he was. *He pushed the medical assistant's hand away when he rubbed Thien's sternum with his knuckles*. Thien had a fast heart rate and low blood pressure, which *fell further when they sat him up*. His feet and hands were quite cold and *when the medical assistant squeezed his fingertip it took three to four seconds for the pink colour to return*. Thien did not have any breathing difficulty.

What could have been the problem with Thien? What would you have done?

Comment   Thien worked in a forested area where there might be malaria. He had non-specific symptoms, including fever which had lasted for two days. On the day he went to the health centre, he had some signs of neurological impairment but was not in coma. He also had a fall in blood pressure when moving from a lying to a sitting position (a postural drop in blood pressure), and delayed capillary refilling, suggesting mild to moderate dehydration. Thien therefore had some of the less clear defining features of severe malaria and was obviously unwell. *If left untreated, he may have become worse rapidly*. Without the aid of a laboratory, a definitive diagnosis of malaria would not be possible, but Thien's symptoms suggest severe malaria. However, other severe infections, including meningitis, should be considered, even though Thien had no obvious neck stiffness.

4 ***Baraka has difficulty breathing***
Baraka is two years old and lives in an area where malaria is especially common at the end of the rainy season. His mother took him to the outpatient department of the local hospital because he had suffered from a *fever and cough* for two days. On the day they went to hospital, she also thought he was a *little short of breath*. The medical attendant at the hospital examined Baraka and found him to be *slightly pale with a fast respiratory rate* (56 breaths per minute). He also had slight *hepatomegaly* but was *alert and not particularly distressed*. The medical attendant thought Baraka probably had a lower respiratory infection, but also considered the possibility of malaria, so gave him an antibiotic and an anti-malarial and sent him home.

The following day Baraka's mother brought him back to the hospital because of *increased difficulty with his breathing*. The medical attendant examining Baraka noted that he had a fast respiratory rate, *nasal flaring and that he was breathing deeply as though he had just been running very fast*. He was pale, still alert but *was unable to sit up by himself*.

What do you think was wrong with Baraka? Why?

Comment   Baraka had extremely common symptoms and signs. Initially, he had no particular signs of severe disease, but his rapid respiratory rate suggested that he might have pneumonia, for which he was appropriately treated. Since malaria is also a common cause of the same symptoms, and in view of the local, high prevalence of malaria, treatment for this possibility was also given. The following day Baraka had developed symptoms consistent with a diagnosis of severe malaria: nasal flaring, deep breathing and prostration. Other diagnoses are also possible, such as pneumonia with septicaemia, but at this stage he clearly needs admission to hospital and laboratory investigations to look for *falciparum* malaria and, if possible, to measure the haemoglobin. The fact that he had already started treatment for malaria does not exclude the possibility that he has developed severe disease.

Parasitological diagnosis

Clinical diagnosis of malaria is unreliable for several reasons.

- Symptoms vary. Although fever is generally present in a patient with malaria, other symptoms and signs may range from mild to severe.
- The clinical features are not specific. The specificity of fever as a symptom of malaria depends upon the causes of febrile illness in

the local population. Other causes such as dengue and typhoid may be more common.

- Other diseases may also be present (see Making a differential diagnosis, page 49).

When a patient's clinical features indicate malaria, the only way to be certain of the diagnosis is to demonstrate that there are malaria parasites in the patient's blood. Wider ranges of laboratory diagnostic procedures are also important in the diagnosis of severe malaria.

Laboratory diagnostic tests:

- confirm the presence of parasites in the blood of symptomatic patients
- confirm complications of severe malaria and assess their severity
- exclude other possible causes of severe disease.

The role of the laboratory in the diagnosis of uncomplicated malaria is to confirm the presence of malaria parasites in the peripheral blood of the patient.

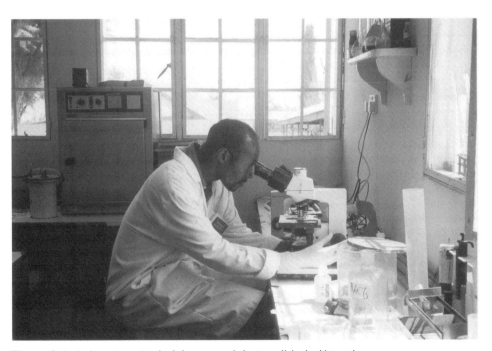

Figure 3.1: Laboratory technician examining a slide in Uganda

In areas of low malaria endemicity, this is often enough to be reasonably confident that the presence of the parasites is the reason for the symptoms seen. However, in areas of high endemicity, this is not so. Finding the parasite is only one of the steps in malaria diagnosis, because infection does not necessarily imply disease, and clinical judgement is always required.

Laboratory confirmation helps to:

- identify patients that need anti-malarial treatment
- reduce unnecessary use of anti-malarial drugs for patients without malaria
- identify malaria species
- identify treatment failures.

Laboratory tests and severe malaria

The basic minimum investigations recommended for patients admitted to hospital for severe malaria should include:

- blood smear for malaria parasites
- haematocrit/haemoglobin level
- blood sugar level
- lumbar puncture in an unconscious patient: where this is not possible give antibiotics for meningitis
- urinalysis for:
  - sugar, to exclude diabetes
  - protein, to exclude pregnancy-induced hypertension

In hospitals where the facilities are available, more comprehensive investigations can be carried out, such as:

- electrolytes and urea – in dehydrated patients
- blood culture – to exclude septicaemia
- chest x-ray – for pulmonary oedema.

Overview of laboratory diagnostic methods for malaria

There are several methods for demonstrating the presence of malaria parasites in peripheral blood, although some of these are used mainly as research tools. Other methods are widely used in malaria endemic and epidemic countries at various levels of the health system. Methods available for demonstrating parasites in blood include:

- light microscopy of stained blood films
- rapid diagnostic test (RDT)
- fluorescence microscopy
- serological diagnosis.

Light microscopy of stained blood films

Light microscopy for malaria parasites using a stained blood film is still the 'gold **standard**' technique for demonstrating the presence of malaria parasites in peripheral blood. It is the most commonly used diagnostic laboratory tool in malaria endemic regions. Two kinds of blood film are used in routine malaria microscopy: thick film and thin film.

Thick film

A thick blood film is made by smearing a large drop of blood over a small area of a slide and allowing it to dry. Any parasites present in the blood are concentrated on the slide. The film is not fixed with methyl alcohol, and therefore when Giemsa stain is added, the red blood cells (RBCs) are lysed (the haemoglobin is removed). A thick film will contain about 20 times more RBCs than a thin film, which makes it quicker and easier to find parasites. However, it is not easy, nor is it recommended, to identify different parasite species using thick films.

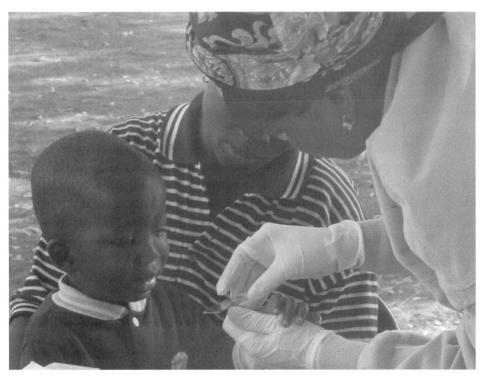

Figure 3.2: Making a malaria blood slide: note the technician wears rubber gloves

Thin film

A thin blood film is made by spreading a small drop of blood over a larger area of the slide, using the edge of another slide. This gives an area with a single layer of RBCs. Fixing the films and staining them with Giemsa allows the parasites to be seen within the RBCs. The use of thin films is recommended for the identification of different species of malaria parasite.

Rapid diagnostic tests

Rapid diagnostic tests (RDTs) are based on the detection of malaria parasite **antigens** in lysed blood, using immunochromatographic methods which are visualised on a dipstick, test strip or test card. A drop of blood is placed on the test strip or card. When the test is positive, the antigens will be fixed by antibody on the test strip. An indicator dye then produces a visible coloured line, in addition to a second 'control' band. Quality control is important for RDTs, as is careful storage, as they are sensitive to humidity. The main types of RDT are:

• Those that detect histidine rich protein-II (HRP-II). This antigen is produced by *P. falciparum*, so this is the only species detected. In some brands of the test, a second line of antibodies is added to detect other species, although with lower sensitivity.
• Those that detect the parasite enzyme lactate dehydrogenase (pLDH) from all four *Plasmodium* species that infect humans. These tests can distinguish *P. falciparum* from other species, but cannot distinguish between *P. vivax*, *P. ovale* and *P. malariae*.

Fluorescence microscopy

Fluorescence microscopy can be used to identify malaria parasites in peripheral blood by the quantitative buffy coat (QBC) technique. This involves the direct staining of thick and thin blood films, using a fluorescent stain called acridine orange. In the QBC technique, blood is centrifuged in a microhaematocrit tube containing acridine orange, and then examined using a fluorescence microscope. If malaria parasites are present, they will be seen as fluorescent bodies at different levels of the sedimentation column, depending upon species and the development stage of the parasite. Although quicker to perform than standard microscopy, fluorescence microscopy is very expensive because it requires specialised equipment, including a fluorescence microscope.

Serological diagnosis

Serological methods detect anti-malaria antibodies mainly through the techniques of indirect fluorescent antibody tests (IFAT) and enzyme linked immunosorbent assay (ELISA). The main use of serological tests is for epidemiological studies. Serological tests cannot distinguish between current and past infection because they detect antibodies. They are not therefore useful as a tool for determining the need for treatment of malaria.

A broad comparison of the main methods as described above is presented in Table 3.4 on page 70.

Methods for detecting malaria parasites in blood at district level

The methods most widely used and most appropriate for diagnosis at district level are microscopic analysis of stained blood films and RDTs. For step-by-step methods of detecting malaria parasites in blood, contact your nearest reference laboratory so that there is local standardisation of methods. If this is not possible, then use standard laboratory procedures, such as those presented in the *Medical Laboratory Manual for Tropical Countries* by M Cheesbrough (1991) and the WHO Benchaids.

Microscopic analysis of stained blood films

The appearance of the four malaria parasite species differs in thick and thin blood films.

Thick film

- There are no red blood cells in thick films (due to haemolysis when stain is added), so the parasites are seen separately on the slide.
- Both the parasites and the white blood cells appear smaller on thick films than on thin films.
- Look for the presence of any yellowish or brown-black pigment, as this is often a good indicator of parasites.
- Trophozoite morphology (see Chapter 1) gives the greatest diagnostic clues to species, as does the number of merozoites in mature schizonts.
- Gametocytes, other than the crescents of *P. falciparum*, look very similar.

Table 3.4: Comparison of main methods for parasitological diagnosis of malaria

Method	Light microscopy: thick film	Light microscopy: thin film	RDTs	Serological
Collecting blood	Children: finger or heel prick Adults: finger prick	Children: finger or heel prick Adults: finger prick	Children: finger or heel prick Adults: finger prick	Children: venous blood or finger or heel prick onto paper. Adults: venous blood or finger prick onto paper
Preparing blood	Giemsa stain, Field's stain	Giemsa stain, Field's stain	Mix with buffer containing haemolysing agent and labelled antibody	Separation of serum from cells or elution from filter paper using physiological saline
How it works	Removes haemoglobin from the blood, concentrates parasites and stains them	Stains malaria parasites within red blood cells	Monoclonal and polyclonal antibodies linked to colour reagents show presence of histidine rich protein-II (HRP-II) or parasite enzyme lactate dehydrogenase (pLDH)	Antibody in patient's blood attaches to malaria antigen on a slide or micro-titre plate and is visualised using an antibody attached to a fluorescent or enzyme linked colour agent
Uses	Confirms presence of malaria parasites; estimates number of infected red blood cells (parasitaemia)	Identifies species of malaria; estimates number of infected red blood cells (parasitaemia)	Diagnosis of *P. falciparum*; identifies a unique protein (HRP-II) inside the red blood cell	Diagnosis of malaria for epidemiological studies: to exclude malaria in cases of fever of unknown cause
Costs	Cheap	Cheap	15–20 times more expensive than blood film diagnosis	Relatively expensive
Notes	The 'gold standard' diagnostic test for malaria		Commercial kits available	

Thin film

- Malaria parasites inside red blood cells have a cytoplasm that stains blue and a small nuclear area that stains a reddish colour.
- More mature parasites can be detected by the presence of yellowish-brown to black pigment.
- As the parasite grows in the red cell, it divides into up to 24 infective schizonts. Some trophozoites differentiate into male and female gametocytes.

Table 3.5 below summarises the parasite stages present and the characteristics of red blood cells in infections with the four different species of malaria parasite.

Table 3.5: Summary of the parasite stages present and the characteristics of red blood cells in infections with the four different species of malaria parasite

	P. falciparum	*P. vivax*	*P. ovale*	*P. malariae*
Parasite stages	usually only young trophozoites and gametocytes seen	all stages of parasite development may be seen	all stages of parasite development may be seen	all stages of parasite development may be seen
Red blood cells	may be many parasites present. RBCs normal or smaller, may have Maurer's clefts (blue dots)	fewer parasites present (usually < 2%). RBCs enlarged, Schüffner's dots and James's dots (stain pink)	usually < 1% of RBCs infected. RBCs enlarged, Schüffner's dots and James's dots (stain pink)	usually < 2% of RBCs become infected. RBCs normal or smaller

NOTE: If you do not find parasites in either thick or thin blood films, report as 'no malaria parasites found,' never as negative. In cases where clinical symptoms suggest malaria, repeat films every eight hours until a diagnosis of some kind is made.

Parasite count on positive slides

After examining the slides and identifying the parasites present, carry out a parasite count. Parasite counts:

- provide an indication of the severity of infection
- indicate how the parasite is responding to drug treatment and help to identify resistance problems.

Parasites may be counted on either thick or thin blood films. It takes practice to become proficient in either method.

Thick film method

This method gives a parasite count per micro-litre (µl) of blood. The number of parasites in a thick blood film is counted in relation to the number of white blood cells (WBCs). A standard WBC count of 8000 per µl of blood is assumed.

1 Count the number of malaria parasites and record the number of WBCs in each field. Continue until you have counted 200 WBCs. If you count ten or more parasites when you have counted 200 WBCs, record the parasite number per 200 WBCs.
2 If you have counted less than ten parasites after reaching 200 WBCs, continue to count parasites until you reach 500 WBCs. Record the parasite number per 500 WBCs.
3 Calculate the parasite count per µl using the following simple formula:

$$\frac{\text{number of parasites counted}}{\text{number of white blood cells}} \times 8000 = \text{parasites per µl}$$

For example, if you have counted 50 parasites and 200 WBCs in the same field divide 50 by 200 and multiply by 8000, which gives a figure of 2000 parasites per µl.

You should count all species present, and then record the asexual stages separately from the gametocytes of *P. falciparum*.

Thin film method

This method is simpler and quicker than the thick film method and expresses the parasite count or infection as a percentage. It gives an approximate guide to severity of infection and **efficacy** of treatment.

1 Select a part of the thin film where the RBCs are lying as a single layer and just touching each other. Count the RBCs and the number of parasite-infected cells in the field using the ×100 objective. Count each infected cell once only as it does not matter how many parasites are in the cell.
2 Continue to do this until you have counted 2000 RBCs, and record the total number of infected cells. Record gametocytes separately from asexual stages.

3 Calculate the percentage parasitaemia as follows:

$$\frac{\text{number of infected red cells}}{2000} \times 100 = \text{percentage parasitaemia}$$

For example, if you have counted 100 infected cells out of 2000 RBCs, divide 100 by 2000 and multiply by 100 to give 5% percentage parasitaemia.

Quality control

It is essential that you have a quality control system to ensure that the results produced in the laboratory are accurate. An incorrect result may mislead the clinician and result in either unnecessary treatment, or cause a delay in treatment which could have serious outcomes.

Internal quality control

Quality control is necessary at each stage of the process of making, reading and interpreting the results of blood microscopy of malaria parasites. The following checks should be part of any internal quality control system.

- The quality of the reagents used: check the pH of the reagents weekly; run known positive controls each time a new batch of stain is made or opened, or every two weeks.
- Quality of staining: pick out slides at random and examine the quality of the stain.
- Cleanliness: ensure that the microscope is cleaned regularly and that the slides used are free from dust or particles that can interfere with microscopy.
- Labelling: are all slides appropriately labelled?
- Reading: use a system of routinely cross-checking the reading of a proportion of positive and negative slides among the microscopists in the laboratory. This may also be extended to parasite counts on positive samples.
- Clerical errors may also be an important source of incorrect results. Try to minimise the transfer of results from worksheets to reporting formats.

External quality assurance

- If an external quality assurance scheme is available, join it. These schemes will periodically send slides for interpretation to participating laboratories. The proportion of correct responses for each participating laboratory will then be circulated. (Laboratories will usually have their own participating code number so that outcomes are confidential.)

- If there are no established schemes, consider setting up a system of quality assurance with neighbouring laboratories, or laboratories in neighbouring districts.
- Cross-checking and supervisory visits are important.

Rapid diagnostic tests

Rapid diagnostic tests are supplied in the form of a commercial kit, which usually will contain all the reagents needed to conduct the test. These normally include:

- buffer solution containing a haemolysing compound, plus a specific antibody labelled with a marker.
- test strip containing a line of capture antibody specific to the antigen under investigation. These may be mixed lines or separate lines of antigens, depending upon the design of the kit. The test strip will also contain a control antibody that will capture the labelled antibody whether attached to an antigen or not.

Where instructions are supplied with the kit, follow these. Figure 3.3 outlines the general type of procedure for such kits.

Comparison of microscopy and rapid diagnostic tests

Ideally, all suspected cases of malaria would be confirmed by microscopy performed by a skilled microscopist. However, there are many areas where such microscopy is not available. RDTs may be useful in some areas and in certain circumstances where microscopy is not available. The relative role of microscopy and RDTs varies, depending upon the level of malaria endemicity in an area. The attributes and roles of each are presented in Table 3.6.

In areas with high transmission rates (mostly in sub-Saharan Africa), the role of microscopy has been limited by inadequate health systems. It is also less helpful to detect parasites in areas where prevalence is high and often not associated with illness. The use of RDTs has been limited to date, but is increasing significantly with the introduction of new drugs. Laboratory confirmation has a use in verifying suspected cases of severe malaria, suspected treatment failures, private sector care and drug resistance. The use of both microscopy and RDTs may need to expand to ensure rational use of more costly treatments.

In low transmission areas, where there are relatively few malaria cases and/or where health staff may not be skilled in malaria microscopy, RDTs may provide an effective alternative to microscopy for the diagnosis of malaria. However, if it is important to

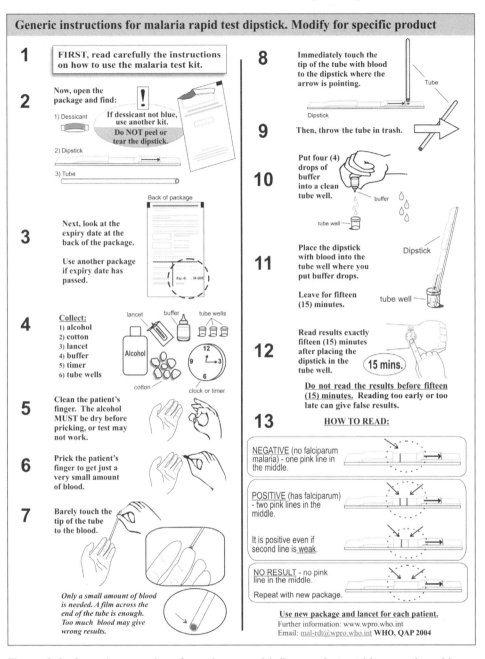

Figure 3.3: Generic procedure for using a rapid diagnostic test kit reproduced by permission of WHO/WPRO

distinguish the species of malaria and confirm all non-*falciparum* cases (because of different treatment **protocols** and the need to prevent relapses with *P. vivax* or *P. ovale*), then it is necessary to use microscopy. This need depends upon the pattern of infecting parasites in the area. In many parts of sub-Saharan Africa, the majority of malaria cases are due to *P. falciparum*, whereas in much of Southeast and South Asia, *P. vivax* also plays a major role so it is more important to identify the infecting species.

Table 3.6: Comparison of the attributes and uses of light microscopy and rapid diagnostic tests (RDTs) in the detection of malaria parasites

	Light microscopy	Rapid diagnostic tests (RDTs)
Sensitivity (the probability that a true positive will be detected)	Dependent upon the ability of the microscopist: skilled microscopists can detect as few as 5–10 parasites per μl of blood; with less skilled microscopists, sensitivity may fall to 100 parasites per μl of blood.	> 90% detection of *P. falciparum* at densities at or above 100 parasites per μl blood; below this level, sensitivity decreases greatly.
Specificity (the probability that *only* true positives will be detected)	Skilled microscopist – approaches 100%	Usually >90%
Detects		
Presence of parasites	Only those in the peripheral circulation	Yes – may also detect parasites in the deep tissues, and in the placenta of pregnant women
Species of parasite	Can distinguish all species	Can detect *P. falciparum* but cannot distinguish *P. vivax*, *P. malariae* or *P. ovale*
Mixed infections	Yes	No
Parasite stages	All	No
Numbers of parasites	Yes	No
Direct cost	US$0.12 to $0.40 per slide examined	US$0.60 to $2.50
Use		
Assessments of malaria prevalence	Yes	Yes
Monitoring of therapy	Yes	No – HRPII tests remain positive 7–14 days or longer after there are no parasites remaining in the blood. pLDH tests can be used.

	Light microscopy	Rapid diagnostic tests (RDTs)
Confirm treatment failure due to resistance	Yes	No – HRPII tests remain positive 7–14 days after there are no parasites remaining in the blood
Prognosis	Yes	No, because are not quantitative
Therapeutic efficacy trials	Yes	No
Emergencies	Usually difficult to find enough skilled microscopists	Yes
Skills and resources required		
Level of skills required	Sensitivity very dependent upon the skills of the microscopist	Requires much less training than for microscopy– but there may be a tendency to underestimate training requirements
Level of resources required	Can use microscope with mirrors – but sensitivity likely to be increased with the use of an electric microscope	No requirement for electricity or special equipment

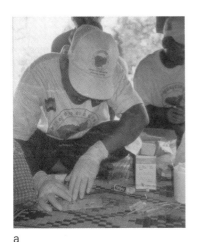
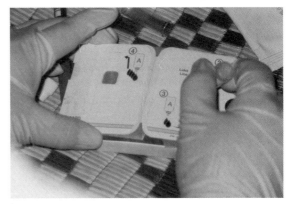

a   b

Figure 3.4a and b: Using a rapid diagnostic test (RDT), Cambodia

Key points

> ▶ Early and accurate diagnosis is extremely important to ensure effective treatment of malaria and to detect other causes of disease.
>
> ▶ Malaria diagnosis should include clinical judgement, based on symptoms and signs, supported by parasitological diagnosis (where facilities allow).
>
> ▶ Clinical judgement should rapidly assess whether the malaria is uncomplicated or severe, so that appropriate treatment can begin as soon as possible.
>
> ▶ Malaria shares symptoms with several other infectious diseases, so taking a careful medical history and conducting a physical examination are important.
>
> ▶ Clinical judgement should rapidly assess whether the malaria is uncomplicated or severe, so that appropriate treatment can begin as soon as possible.
>
> ▶ Laboratory diagnosis is important to: confirm presence of parasites in the blood of symptomatic patients, confirm complications and assess their severity, exclude other possible causes of severe disease.
>
> ▶ The most important methods for parasitological diagnosis are light microscopy of stained blood films and rapid diagnostic tests (RDTs).

Further reading

1   Mturi N. et al (2003) 'Cerebral malaria – optimising management', CNS Drugs 17(3): 153–165
2   'Severe *falciparum* malaria', Transactions of the Royal Society of Tropical Medicine and Hygiene 94 Suppl 1:S1–90, WHO, 2000
3   *Management of Severe Malaria: a practical handbook*, WHO, 2000, second edition
4   Cheesbrough, M. *District Laboratory Practice in Tropical Countries*, Part 1 and Part 2, Cambridge University Press, 2005 and 2006, second edition (Part 1 also available through TALC [Teaching-aids At Low Cost])

4 ▶ The Treatment of Malaria

Mike English

This chapter describes:

▶ the principles and procedures of malaria management

▶ the management of uncomplicated malaria and associated conditions

▶ clinical features indicating treatment failure and possible reasons

▶ resistance to anti-malarial drugs

▶ the management of severe malaria and associated conditions

▶ the management of malaria at the periphery, including the Integrated Management of Childhood Illness (IMCI) and home care

▶ delivery systems for case management.

It will be useful for those responsible for the treatment of malaria at different levels of health facility. It will also be helpful for health managers who need to understand the system requirements for treating malaria effectively.

Introduction

The treatment of malaria varies according to the geographical location in which it occurs, according to national guidelines and according to the drugs available within a particular country or region. The development of resistance to anti-malarial drugs means that treatment policies are under constant review and subject to change. In this chapter we describe the current principles and procedures of malaria management, which aim both to prevent death from malaria and to reduce severe illness.

Principles of malaria management

The most important principles of malaria management are:

- early and accurate diagnosis
- prompt and effective treatment
- good nursing care
- **adherence** to treatment
- advice and **follow-up**.

By following these principles you could help to reduce treatment failures, decrease the number of patients who become severely or dangerously ill, reduce the number who die and delay the development of drug resistance in your area.

Decisions about the approach to malaria treatment depend on:

- the species of malaria parasite
- the severity of illness
- the availability of drugs and facilities for treatment
- levels of anti-malarial drug resistance locally
- prior treatment received by the patient.

Early and accurate diagnosis

The level of early and accurate diagnosis will depend upon how promptly your patients seek diagnosis and treatment when they have symptoms, and how quickly patients are seen by the appropriate people when they come to hospital (i.e. patient triage). It will also depend on the quality of the diagnosis they receive when they present for consultation.

Factors that influence when and where a patient presents with symptoms of malaria vary in different locations and in differing socio-economic groups. They include:

- knowledge and beliefs about illness and treatment in general and malaria in particular
- experiences, perceptions and attitudes towards illness and treatment, including experience of particular providers and/or certain drugs
- quality and cost of care
- access to providers and/or treatment (including geographical, social and economic access).

Information, education and communication (IEC) activities are intended to promote an understanding within communities of the need for early diagnosis and the importance of presenting for treatment at a health facility. They are an important intervention for increasing early access to health facilities.

In malaria endemic countries, the equipment and trained personnel necessary for laboratory diagnosis are often not available in health facilities and diagnostic decisions have to be made on clinical presentations (symptoms and signs) alone. As discussed in Chapter 3: Clinical and Parasitological Diagnosis of Malaria, the clinical presentation of malaria is often similar to that of other diseases and this can make diagnosis difficult. Health personnel have to make urgent decisions about treatment when faced with a non-specific illness that might or might not be malaria. For many first level workers, the Integrated Management of Childhood Illness (IMCI) strategy provides a solution to the problems of making an accurate diagnosis of malaria on clinical presentation alone. The IMCI approach stresses the need to identify appropriate treatment quickly without necessarily reaching a diagnosis. It uses clinical **algorithms** to classify children by the treatment they require. The classification may cover a range of clinical conditions, but the immediate priority is that the child receives the treatment he or she requires. A specific diagnosis can be made at the referral level if required. The IMCI approach is described in more detail on page 113.

Box 4.1: Key steps before providing malaria treatment

Step 1
Identify patients who have severe disease or are at risk of complications, and those from high risk groups.

Step 2
Find out what previous treatment, if any, the patient has taken and whether or not they are able to take oral medication.

Step 3
Make an accurate diagnosis within the limits of the facilities available to you.

Step 4
Determine whether the patient should be treated or referred immediately.

Step 5
In cases of malaria with severe complications, it is particularly important to determine:
- the degree of neurological impairment or coma
- the need for immediate intravenous fluids or blood transfusion
- whether hypoglycaemia is present.

Prompt and effective treatment

Appropriate treatment of malaria can save lives. Prompt and effective treatment reduces the duration of malarial disease and prevents the development of complications. As with early and accurate diagnosis, it is vital that patients seek treatment quickly once they are aware of symptoms and that health workers act fast. IEC activities have an important role in promoting prompt treatment.

District managers (or their equivalent) need to decide how best to use the resources available at each level of health facility in order to ensure the most prompt and effective treatment. However, in general and where conditions permit, a severely ill patient, especially one who is comatose, should be managed in an intensive care unit or the highest level of referral facility.

Effectiveness of treatment

Effectiveness of treatment depends upon:
- efficacy of the drug (see section on Resistance to anti-malarials, page 89)
- health personnel using anti-malarial drugs correctly and following treatment guidelines (see National treatment guidelines, page 84)
- adherence to the treatment (see opposite).

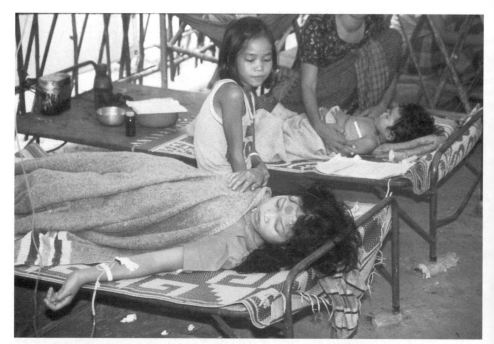

Figure 4.1: Treatment of a woman with malaria on the Thai-Cambodia border

Many people who live in malaria endemic areas do not have access to good information about malaria treatment and prevention, or to effective and affordable anti-malarials. In some countries, the majority of people with febrile illness will buy medicines from retail outlets. It is only when their symptoms continue, or become more severe, that they present for consultation at a health centre. In order to achieve the goals of early and accurate diagnosis, as well as prompt and effective treatment in all cases of malaria, more work needs to be done to educate the people involved. Community and retail drug sellers need to be aware of the importance of early diagnosis and treatment and the symptoms that point to severe malaria (see Home care and management, page 121).

Adherence to treatment

'Adherence' is carrying out the advice given by a doctor or other health care provider, in other words, abiding by their recommendations on both drug regimen and dosage. Encouraging adherence is very important. Factors which influence whether or not a patient will adhere to a drug regimen include:

- how long the treatment lasts
- the number of daily doses
- how quickly a response to treatment is seen, particularly in the reduction of fever side effects
- affordability or price in relation to **household** income
- presentation and packaging
- health education messages
- the size of the tablet and its taste and/or colour
- perceptions of the drug due to its reputation.

Good nursing care, advice and follow-up

Counselling and follow-up, especially of high-risk groups, are important in encouraging adherence to drug treatment and identifying problems.

When you are prescribing medication, give patients appropriate information. Patients and their families need to understand how much medication they should take and for how long. They also need to see the importance of returning to the health facility if the condition does not improve, becomes worse or if new symptoms develop.

You need to ensure effective follow-up and observation of patients during the illness and during the recovery period. The most important issues in follow-up, observation and nursing care are discussed later in this chapter.

Management of uncomplicated malaria

It is vital that patients are given the best disease management possible in the early stages of their illness. Uncomplicated *falciparum* malaria can progress to severe disease within just a few hours, particularly in children. The disease must be recognised early and effective treatment started quickly; such treatment needs to be available as close to the home as possible.

National treatment guidelines

Most malaria affected countries have a national anti-malarial drug policy and national treatment guidelines. These provide country specific recommendations and regulations on anti-malarial drugs and their use. The guidelines may recommend treatment that is the same throughout the country but, where levels of malaria endemicity vary within different areas of the country, the local treatment policy may vary.

National anti-malarial treatment policies and guidelines provide a framework for the effective treatment of malaria. They commonly include regimens for:

- first-line treatment of probable or confirmed malaria in adults and children
- second and third-line treatment given to treatment failures in adults and children
- treatment of severe malaria in adults and in children
- treatment and protection of pregnant women, including intermittent preventive treatment (see Chapter 6: Malaria in Pregnancy).

Where national treatment guidelines have been formulated they should be followed by all health care providers, both in the public and in the private sectors.

The national treatment policy works within the economic and infrastructure constraints of the country and aims to:

- provide a rapid **clinical cure** which is long lasting
- reduce morbidity
- prevent the progression of uncomplicated malaria to severe malaria
- provide protection to pregnant women and their babies (see Chapter 6)
- reduce the rate of development of drug resistance

- in low transmission areas only, reduce transmission through the use of gametocytocidal drugs (see Chapter 2: The Epidemiology of Malaria).

National malaria treatment policy may change as resistance to commonly used anti-malarial drugs, particularly the first-line drug of treatment, develops. It is therefore important to use the current version of the policy. Factors that indicate that the treatment policy needs revising include:

- evidence from therapeutic efficacy studies of increased resistance
- evidence of increased malaria-associated mortality and morbidity
- consumer and provider dissatisfaction with the current policy
- evidence of better drugs, strategies and approaches.

Anti-malarial drugs

When treating uncomplicated malaria, the most commonly used drugs are:

- chloroquine
- sulfadoxine-pyrimethamine (SP)
- amodiaquine
- artemisinin and its derivatives (mainly artesunate and artemether)
- combinations of artemisinin derivatives with other drugs, such as lumefantrine or amodiaquine – known as Artemisinin-based Combination Therapies or ACT.

Less commonly used for uncomplicated malaria are:

- quinine (with tetracycline or doxycycline where there is quinine resistance)
- mefloquine
- halofantrine
- atovaquone-proguanil.

Treatment of *Plasmodium falciparum* malaria and malaria where the species is unknown

WHO recommends that first-line treatment in all countries experiencing resistance to conventional monotherapies (such as chloroquine, SP and amodiaquine) should use combination therapies, preferably those containing artemisinin derivatives. Many countries are now adopting such a change in policy. This is because of their high efficacy, very rapid **parasite** and symptom **clearance times** and strong effect on reducing gametocyte carriage rate, which helps to reduce the transmission of resistance. As the value of artemisinin derivatives is so great, it is important to ration their use to prevent resistance from developing.

Administer first-line drugs orally. Use second-line drugs only in cases of treatment failure, where a patient is allergic or intolerant to the first-line drug, or where the first-line drug is contraindicated.

The Annex at the end of this chapter (pages 126–141) provides schedules for the most commonly used drugs and details of any adverse effects they may cause. However, *where national treatment guidelines are in place, they should be followed.*

Treatment of non-*falciparum* infections

Treatment with chloroquine is the standard recommended therapy for malaria caused by *P. vivax*, *P. malariae* and *P. ovale*. In areas of chloroquine sensitivity, a three-day course of treatment kills most stages of all the non-*falciparum* species. However, chloroquine does not kill the liver stages (hypnozoites) of *P. vivax* or *P. ovale*. For this, you will need an additional drug, primaquine. In some areas, especially where transmission is not intense, treatment with primaquine is routinely indicated to prevent relapse of *P. vivax* infections. The regimen needed for this **radical cure** depends upon the parasites' sensitivity to primaquine, which differs by area. For example, for strains of *P. vivax* from Papua New Guinea, the Solomon Islands and Vanuatu, and parts of Indonesia, 30 mg of primaquine base daily for fourteen days is required for a complete cure.

Malaria in pregnant women

Anti-malarials recommended for both the treatment and prevention of malaria in pregnancy are discussed in Chapter 6. Several drugs used for treatment of malaria are contraindicated in pregnancy.

Combination therapy

Combination therapy with anti-malarial drugs is the use of two or more blood schizonticidal drugs which act independently of each other and have different biochemical targets in the parasite. CTs are divided into artemisinin-based combinations (ACT) and non-artemisinin-based combinations. ACTs are the preferred choice. CT does not include:

• multiple drug therapies where a non-anti-malarial is used to increase the effect of the anti-malarial

- drugs such as sulfadoxine-pyrimethamine (S-P) where the individual drugs could not be used to treat malaria.

Co-formulated CTs are manufactured together in the same tablet or capsule. *Co-administered* CTs are separate tablets or capsules of each drug, given at the same time. Because the patient could take just one of the drugs in a co-administered CT, they are more likely to be misused than co-formulated CTs. However, the use of blister packaging with the co-administered drugs kept together, is likely to improve adherence.

There are two aims in the use of combination therapies (CT):

- to improve the efficacy of the therapy by using two drugs instead of one
- to delay the development of resistance to each of the individual drugs in the combination.

How well a CT achieves both of these aims depends on the level of resistance to the drugs in the combination that already exists *before* they are combined. Where there is already a high level of resistance, the protection will be lower.

The following operational constraints need to be overcome to make the best use of CTs:

- affordability – they are relatively expensive
- acceptability to patients, providers and policy makers
- adherence by patients
- access through public and private sectors
- use in pregnancy.

Combination drugs under development, where the initial evidence of efficacy is promising, are:

- chlorproguanil/dapsone combined with artesunate
- a fixed dose combination of piperaquine and dihydroartemisinin (DHA)
- a combination of pyronaridine and artesunate or DHA.

Management of conditions associated with uncomplicated malaria

The three important ancillary treatments in cases of uncomplicated malaria are

- rehydration
- fever (**hyperpyrexia**) reduction
- treatment of anaemia.

Rehydration

Assess dehydration, especially in children, and treat with oral rehydration salts. Advise all patients to drink plenty of fluids, and advise families to continue giving fluids and food to young children, including continuing to breastfeed.

Hyperpyrexia

Hyperpyrexia is a rectal temperature of more than 40° C or an axillary temperature of more than 39.5° C. It can affect the patient's mental status and may cause some to vomit, making it difficult for them to take oral medications. Anti-pyretics should be given to patients with hyperpyrexia before any other drugs, especially to children who may be at risk of febrile seizures. Steps in managing hyperpyrexia are as follows:

- remove as much clothing as possible
- fan the patient and cool with tepid sponging. Recent studies, however, suggest these may be ineffective
- give an anti-pyretic drug, such as paracetamol, by mouth or as a suppository. Alternatively, give syrup or crushed tablets via a nasogastric tube.

Note: Do not give aspirin to children under twelve years of age.

Anaemia

Pregnant women and children under five are at the greatest risk of developing anaemia as a result of *P. falciparum* and *P. vivax* malaria. Anaemia can reduce the effectiveness of malaria treatment, especially in children in Africa, so it is extremely important to diagnose and treat anaemia as early as possible.

Treatment failure

Treatment failure is defined as 'the failure to clear malaria parasites effectively from the blood, with a reappearance of symptoms within days or weeks of the initial anti-malarial treatment'. Clinical features that indicate a failure of treatment include:

- clinical deterioration
- slow clinical response
- reappearance of previously resolved clinical symptoms
- chronic anaemia secondary to repeated parasitaemia.

It is important to remember that *while drug resistance can cause treatment failure, not all treatment failure is due to drug resistance.* There are a number of reasons why treatment may have failed:

- misdiagnosis – the illness was not malaria
- the patient has another fever-causing illness in addition to malaria
- the patient did not take the full dose of the drug
- the wrong dose of drug was prescribed
- the effectiveness of the anti-malarial has been reduced by interaction with another drug
- the drug was of poor quality and contained low concentrations of active anti-malarial
- the drug was poorly absorbed, for example due to vomiting
- the patient has been re-infected with malaria or another fever-causing illness.

How you deal with treatment failure will depend on the cause of the failure.

Resistance to anti-malarials

Anti-malarial drug resistance is increasing. It has led to a significant loss of efficacy of the most affordable and commonly used anti-malarial drugs. It has been a major problem in countries such as Thailand, Myanmar and Cambodia in Southeast Asia, where there is now multi-drug resistance. Drug resistance is also spreading elsewhere. Several sub-Saharan African countries have reported high failure rates for chloroquine when used to treat *P. falciparum* malaria. As a result, these countries have changed their policy on first-line drugs. Resistance to sulfadoxine-pyrimethamine is also rising in sub-Saharan Africa, particularly in the East.

The implications of resistance to anti-malarial drugs are immense. Many malaria endemic countries are beginning to have no affordable, effective anti-malarial drugs available. The cost of changing to newer, more expensive anti-malarial drugs for treatment could overwhelm the limited health budgets of most of the countries in sub-Saharan Africa.

Resistance to anti-malarials has been described for both *P. falciparum* and *P. vivax*. *P. falciparum* resistance to nearly every anti-malarial in use has been reported somewhere in the world. There have been reports of *P. vivax* resistance to chloroquine and primaquine in limited areas. Chloroquine resistant *P. vivax* is not

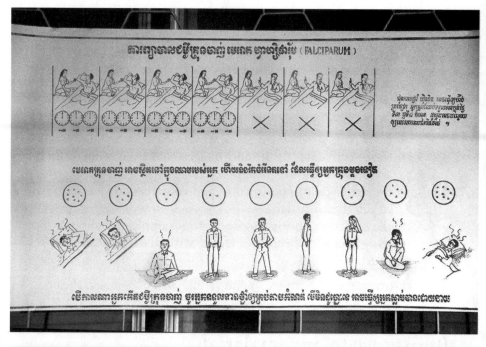

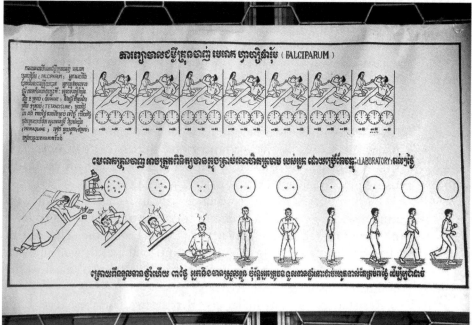

Figure 4.2: Education posters from Cambodia:

a   shows the effects of not taking the full course of treatment – in this case only four out of seven days. Parasites and symptoms return.

b   shows the benefits of completing the full course of treatment.

yet a major public health problem. This is because it occurs mainly in areas with intense transmission where most patients are semi-immune, so that chloroquine still has acceptable effectiveness. Quinine resistance is still rare in Africa, but is increasing in South East Asia.

How is drug resistance defined?

Anti-malarial drug resistance can be defined in terms of parasito-logical responses *and* clinical responses. Parasitological failure is when a drug fails to remove parasites from the bloodstream for a defined period of time. Clinical failure is when the drug fails to clear signs and symptoms in a defined time. Parasitological and clinical failure are not necessarily the same. Sometimes, although there is clinical cure, blood films will show that parasitological cure has not been achieved. This may be an adequate response in areas with highly endemic malaria, where the population is generally semi-immune, but not in patients who are non-immune. It is important that all countries monitor response to their first-line treatment regularly through standard tests, in which clinical and parasitological response to treatment with a given drug is followed over a period of 28 days. The classification of response to treatment is shown in Box 4.2.

Box 4.2: Classification of treatment outcomes according to WHO protocol, 2005

Early treatment failure
- Danger signs or severe malaria on Day 1, 2 or 3, in the presence of parasitaemia
- Parasitaemia on Day 2 higher than on Day 0, irrespective of axillary temperature
- Parasitaemia on Day 3 with axillary temperature $\geq$37.5 °C
- Parasitaemia on Day 3 $\geq$25% of count on Day 0

Late clinical failure
- Danger signs or severe malaria in the presence of parasitaemia on any day after Day 4 and before Day 28, without the patient previously meeting any of the criteria of early treatment failure
- Axillary temperature $\geq$37.5 °C in the presence of parasitaemia on any day between Day 4 and Day 28, without the patient previously meeting any of the criteria of early treatment failure

Late parasitological failure
- Presence of parasitaemia between Day 7 and Day 28 with temperature <37.5 °C, without the patient previously meeting any of the criteria of early treatment failure or late clinical failure

Adequate clinical and parasitological response
- Absence of parasitaemia on Day 28, irrespective of axillary temperature, without the patient meeting any of the criteria of early treatment failure, late clinical failure or late parasitological failure

(Reproduced from Appendix 1 Methods and Techniques for Clinical Trials on Antimalarial Drug Efficacy: Genotyping to Identify Parasite Populations May 2007. http://apps.who.int/malaria/docs/drugresistance/malariaGenotyping.pdf ISBN 9789241596305 by permission of the WHO)

How does drug resistance develop and spread?

Anti-malarial drugs target specific proteins in the malaria parasite. It is possible for the genes producing these proteins or genes controlling access of the drug to the parasite to mutate spontaneously. If this happens, the anti-malarial drug will no longer be effective. The number of different mutations needed for the parasite to become resistant varies with different drugs – some need only a single mutation, while others need several. These resistant parasites will survive, whilst those that are still drug sensitive will be killed by the drug.

A few parasites will always manage to survive treatment with anti-malarials. These are normally removed by the immune system. The specific immune response in people who have semi-immunity to malaria is likely to clear parasites more efficiently than the non-specific immune response (in non-immunes). This has been proposed as a reason for the rapid rate of development of resistance in South East Asia where the majority of the population is non-immune.

Resistance may develop more quickly to drugs which have a long half-life (that stay in the bloodstream for a long time). There will be levels of the drug in the bloodstream that are high enough to exert selective pressure on the parasites, but not high enough to eliminate them. It is thought that under these conditions, resistant mutations will spread. On the other hand, these long half-life drugs, such as sulfadoxine-pyrimethamine (SP) and mefloquine (MQ), have the advantage that they can be given in simple, single dose regimens which improve adherence and make it possible to observe the therapy directly.

Development of resistance to one drug may facilitate resistance to another drug if they are closely related chemically. This is called cross-resistance. Cross-resistance is known between chloroquine and amodiaquine. Development of resistance to mefloquine may lead to resistance to halofantrine and quinine.

One of the dangers of the use of presumptive treatment for malaria (treatment without confirmed parasitological diagnosis) is that it has the potential to help the development and spread of drug resistance by increasing the number of people who are treated unnecessarily. This is based on some of those people becoming infected, while there is still some level of drug in the body.

How do we recognise the presence of drug resistance?

Drug resistance can be measured using *in vivo* and *in vitro* tests, where facilities are available. Testing procedures are described in WHO (2003) and WHO (2005) – see Further reading, page 124.

In areas with no microscopy or poor quality of results, you may find it difficult to recognise anti-malarial drug resistance. In many of those areas where malaria diagnosis is presumptive, detection of treatment failures is also presumptive.

Case reports or series of case reports

You can use case reports or series of case reports to indicate the presence of treatment failure. These may, however, present a **biased** view since **denominators** (total number of cases) will be unknown and the actual rates of resistance cannot be calculated.

Increased use of second-line drugs

Increased use of second-line drugs may indicate increased numbers of treatment failures, assuming first-line drugs are available and used by prescribers. However, this presumes that many treatment failures are recognised and patients are given second-line drugs, and that most treatment failures are due to drug resistance. In many situations, patients with resistant parasites are not treated with alternative drugs. This may be either because resistance is not detected, or because alternative drugs are not available. Alternatively, clinical relapse can occur after two or three weeks and the patient may go to hospital. It is also possible, during times of intense malaria transmission, that the new symptoms may be classified as a new infection and treated with the same drug as before. This places such patients at higher risk of developing severe disease.

Increase in malaria-associated morbidity and mortality

The development of anti-malarial drug resistance will be accompanied by an increase in malaria-associated mortality and morbidity. In areas where *P. falciparum* is present together with other species, an increase in the **ratio** of *P. falciparum* to the other species may be an indication of increasing drug resistance. Such increases may also be due to an epidemic (in prone areas), migration, over or misdiagnosis, so do not prove increasing resistance.

Preventing the spread of drug resistance

It is very important that district authorities and individual health workers take steps to prevent the spread of resistant strains. You need to ensure that:

- all individual patients take a full course of drug treatment
- health facilities and other outlets follow national policy and guidelines
- the quality of drugs is regulated.

Ensuring that all individual patients take a full course of drug treatment will involve:

- making sure that your patient is given the right dosage of the drug for the right duration
- giving them appropriate advice on how to take it
- trying to make sure that they adhere to the advice.

This, in turn, requires appropriate health education of the community, and training of health workers and others who dispense drugs (see Home care and management, page 121).

Always use the most recent version of national guidelines. These should be disseminated to all health facilities and retailers of anti-malarials. Community health education is also important so that patients and their carers are aware of the national policies on treatment and can make informed decisions when purchasing anti-malarials from untrained distributors.

Drugs may be poor quality due to counterfeiting or poor manufacturing. They may have deteriorated as a result of inappropriate handling and storage, or they may be past their expiry date. Poor quality drugs when taken at dosages recommended by the national guidelines may still facilitate the development of resistance where levels are not sufficient to eliminate parasites. It is the responsibility of national drug regulatory authorities within the ministry of health to assure the quality of anti-malarials and other drugs. District staff need to ensure proper storage and use before expiry.

Re-treatment of suspected treatment failures

National policy on procedures for re-treatment of treatment failures should be part of the national anti-malarial treatment guidelines. You will need to assess the likely reason for failure: this means questioning the patient, as well as using your knowledge of local levels of drug resistance. Options include:

- When you suspect the patient did not receive a full and adequate dose rather than drug resistance, retreat with the same drug ensuring appropriate dosing, adherence and quality of drug. Make sure that no other drugs are being taken by the patient that might cause reduced effectiveness.
- Detect and treat other causes of illness. Where possible, take a malaria blood smear to be sure that the symptoms are due to malaria.
- When you suspect a **recrudescent** infection, treat with the second-line drug as recommended in the national treatment guidelines.
- If the patient has deteriorated clinically and severe malaria is likely, treat as a patient with severe malaria (treat immediately and refer if you are in a peripheral facility).
- If a confirmed P. vivax case fails to respond to chloroquine, you can treat with quinine or mefloquine.

Case studies

1 **Olayemi becomes ill again**

Olayemi is four years old. He was seen at his local health centre a week ago with a two-day history of fever, cough and tiredness. A blood film showed many malaria parasites, and chloroquine in standard doses was prescribed. He improved initially, but two days before returning to the hospital was unwell again with fever and some abdominal pain. Examination found that he had fever and was pale. He *was able to walk and talk,* and had hepatosplenomegaly. A blood smear was taken and showed numerous malaria parasites. The medical attendant diagnosed recrudescent or resistant malaria and prescribed sulfadoxine-pyrimethamine before discharge.

How would you have managed this case?

Comment   Such stories are becoming very common in many African countries where chloroquine resistance is increasing rapidly. However, as this case illustrates, even when the parasites are obviously chloroquine-resistant, the patient may respond to treatment. It is particularly difficult, in areas of intense malaria transmission, for clinicians to decide whether the appearance of malaria symptoms 14–28 days after a course of treatment represents a real relapse or a new infection. Local knowledge of parasite sensitivity to first-line anti-malarial drugs is essential in such situations.

The choice of second-line treatment should reflect regional or national policy. Children who present again should be examined to assess whether they have developed severe disease and require admission. The medical attendant might also have chosen to prescribe oral iron supplements for Olayemi, because he was pale. Observing the child take the medicine, particularly if treating with a 'once only' drug, is advisable. Carers should be advised about the importance of taking a full course of treatment – failure to do this may cause clinical relapse.

2 **Rehema still has a high temperature**

Two year old Rehema presented to hospital with a history of fever and a single convulsion. She had a positive blood smear for malaria and on examination had a *high temperature but otherwise appeared to be well.* She was treated with sulfadoxine-pyrimethamine (Fansidar®) and allowed home. Two days later her mother brought her back saying that she *still had a high fever.* A repeat blood smear still showed a few malaria parasites. The medical attendant advised the mother to buy some halofantrine from the private pharmacy because the child had 'resistant' malaria.

How would you have managed this case?
Comment   Rehema's history is fairly typical of malaria illness in many countries
and she was treated on the basis of new national guidelines. But, she was still
febrile after two days and had a positive blood smear. In this example, the
advice given to her mother may have been inappropriate. Unlike chloroquine,
sulfadoxine-pyrethamine has no anti-pyretic action, so parasitaemia and fever can
take two to three days to clear. If, as in this case, the patient is otherwise well
and the parasitaemia is reduced, it would have been reasonable to wait a further
48 hours before considering the possibility of a resistant infection. Other possible
causes of persistent fever, such as otitis media or salmonella infection, should also
have been eliminated.

3 *Nguyen does not know where he is*
Nguyen, a 24-year-old trainee civil engineer, became ill while working on a
road building project in an area known to have multi-resistant *falciparum*
malaria. He developed a high fever, headaches, and generalised aches and pains,
and was seen at the outpatient department of the nearest hospital. Malaria was
diagnosed on the basis of a blood film, and Nguyen was prescribed oral mefloquine
and artesunate and sent home. Within 24 hours he was brought back to hospital
because he *did not appear to know where he was or to recognise his friends*, and
seemed to be suffering from *intermittent hallucinations*. He was given a sedative
drug by the outpatient doctor and admitted for observation.
How would you have managed this case?

Comment   This example raises several issues. Nguyen may have developed
cerebral malaria, and non-adherence should be investigated as a possible cause.
Alternatively, he may either be experiencing an acute adverse reaction to
mefloquine, or the cause of the problem is not malaria. Nguyen should have been
completely reassessed when he presented again, focusing in particular on other
signs of severe malaria. This reassessment should have included: examination
of a new blood film and, if available, re-examination of the original blood film,
measurement of blood glucose, and laboratory evaluation of renal function if
feasible. Following this, arrangements should have been made for continuation
of treatment, and for close observation. Transfer to a more specialist unit, if
available, might also have been appropriate.

Management of severe malaria

Treat severe malaria as an emergency. Cerebral malaria and severe anaemia are the most common manifestations of severe malaria. Delay in diagnosis and inappropriate treatment, especially in infants and children, can result in rapid deterioration.

The management of severe malaria requires appropriately qualified clinical staff and the facilities of a referral hospital. This section aims to remind staff of the key points in the management of severe malaria.

Box 4.3   Management of severe malaria

Severe malaria should be managed using the following important steps:

1 Start treatment immediately on the basis of clinical presentation. Make a blood film for parasitological confirmation which should be examined as soon as possible. Give anti-malarial drug intravenously or intramuscularly. Give oral treatment as soon as the patient can take oral medication safely. Calculate doses based on weight (mg/kg); this is very important for children.

2 Consider the need for a blood transfusion; in particular if the patient has anaemia that is contributing to respiratory distress or that appears to be life-threatening.

3 Reduce high body temperature if more than 39° C by giving paracetamol by mouth if possible, or alternatively by suppository.

4 Assess fluid requirement and maintain good fluid balance, avoiding over-hydration or under-hydration.

5 Control convulsions, by first correcting any detectable cause such as hypoglycaemia or hyperpyrexia, and give an anti-convulsant drug.

6 Check blood glucose level as soon as possible, give glucose to correct hypoglycaemia, and monitor frequently including rechecking blood glucose after 30 minutes and throughout management of the illness.

7 Treat or exclude other causes of coma.

8 Monitor core temperature, respiration rate, blood pressure, level of consciousness and other vital signs frequently.

9 Monitor therapeutic response frequently, and look for and treat any other infections.

10 Monitor urine output constantly and look for 'black urine'. Decide whether a urinary catheter is necessary, for example if acute renal failure or pulmonary oedema is suspected, to guide fluid balance. Decide also if a central venous pressure line is required, if pulmonary oedema is suspected, or if the patient is in shock or has impending renal failure.
11 Conduct regular laboratory measurements of: haematocrit, glucose, urea or creatinine, and electrolytes. Take blood cultures if a patient goes into shock during treatment.
12 Conduct opthalmoscopic examination of the fundus to check for retinal haemorrhage.

NOTE: More detailed guidelines for the treatment of severe malaria are available in: *Management of Severe Malaria: a practical handbook*, WHO, 2000, second edition. On website: *www.rbm.who.int*

Treatment guidelines for severe malaria

Commonly used drugs for severe malaria are quinine and artemisinin derivatives. Table 4.1 provides treatment guidelines for severe malaria. However, where national treatment guidelines are available these should be followed.

Management of conditions associated with severe malaria

As discussed in Chapter 3, many of the clinical symptoms of severe malaria are similar to those associated with other severe illnesses. Clinical management of severe malaria, therefore, has much in common with clinical management of any seriously ill patient.

Good ancillary treatment and supportive care of patients with severe malaria, which do not require sophisticated health facilities, are also very important in preventing death and disability. Careful follow-up and observation, following initial treatment, is also very important to:

• monitor the patient's progress; signs of recovery are desirable and those of deterioration signal the need for urgent intervention
• control the delivery of drugs and infusion fluids to avoid fluid overload and drug overdoses
• detect early the development of complications, so that their management can be initiated in time to prevent permanent damage or death
• detect any side effects to the drugs being given; if of a serious nature, then change to another suitable drug.

Table 4.1: Treatment of severe malaria

	Hospital, high dependency ward, or Intensive Care Unit	Busy hospital ward or health centre	Rural clinic (no injections possible)
Quinine	Quinine di-hydrochloride 7 mg salt/kg infused over 30 minutes followed by 10 mg/kg over 4 hours Maintenance dose: 10 mg/kg salt infused over 2–4 hours and given 8 hourly	A **loading dose** of Quinine di-hydrochloride 20 mg salt/kg diluted to 60mg/ml with sterile water given in two equal divided doses in the anterolateral part of each thigh (not in the buttock) Maintenance dose 10 mg/kg 8 hourly or 12 hourly in areas of Africa where quinine sensitivity is high	Artemisinin suppositories 10 mg/kg at 0 and 4 hours, then 7 mg/kg at 24, 36, 48 + 60 hours
Artemisinin derivatives (treat for 5–7 days)	Artemether 3.2 mg/kg stat by IM injection followed by 1.6 mg/kg at 24 hour intervals; OR artesunate 2 mg/kg stat by IV injection followed by 1 mg/kg at 12 hours and then 1 mg/kg daily	As for hospital ICU. Artesunate can also be given by IM injection	Artemisinin suppositories 10 mg/kg at 0 and 4 hours followed by 7 mg/kg at 24, 36, 48 and 60 hours

NOTES:
- Infusions of quinine can be given in 10 ml/kg of 0.9% saline, 5% or 10% dextrose.
- Avoid giving a loading dose if there is reliable evidence that the patient received quinine, halofantrine or mefloquinine in the preceding 24 hours. Start with the maintenance dose instead.
- All drug doses must be reduced in established renal failure. Reduce quinine to 5–7 mg/kg in this case and if the patient is on **parenteral** therapy for more than 48 hours.
- Quinine when injected should be given as a deep intramuscular injection. It should never be given subcutaneously. It is important to clean the skin adequately before injecting.
- Oral treatment should start as soon as the patient can swallow well enough to complete a full course of treatment. In some cases this may mean that an alternative drug to quinine can be used to complete the course of treatment, for example, sulfadoxine-pyrimethamine may be given, where there is no SP resistance.
- If an artemisinin suppository is expelled within the first hour, insert another one immediately.

Ministry of Health

Management of the Patient with
SEVERE MALARIA

1. Start resuscitation, particularly maintenance of a patent airway.

2. Establish IV line.

3. Make a thick blood smear for immediate malaria parasite count.

4. Detect and Treat Hypoglycaemia if blood glucose ≤ 2.2mmol/l or ≤ 40mg/dl
Give 1ml/kg of 50% dextrose IV, diluted with an equal volume of 0.9% Saline, given slowly over 3-5 minutes. Follow with 10% dextrose infusion at 5ml/kg/hr.

5. If there is no test for blood glucose, treat as if the patient is Hypoglycaemic.

6. Start Quinine 10mg/kg intravenously:
Quinine should be diluted in 10ml/kg of isotonic fluid (0.9% Saline or 5% Dextrose) for a child or 500mls for an adult. Give quinine IV over 4 hours every 8 hours until the patient can take orally

7. Assess patient's fluid requirements;
Look for signs of fluid depletion or shock (Systolic Bp <50mmHg in children 1-5 yrs or <80 mmHg in >5yrs.).
Rx; 30ml/kg 0.9% Saline IV in 1 hour (NG infusion may be used if IV not possible) then, reassess. Give oxygen if possible.

8. Control fever if the body temperature measured in the axillae is 38.5°C and above: Rx Oral or rectal Paracetamol (15mg/kg every 4 to 6 hours). Tepid sponge and fan the patient.

9. Control convulsions if there are 3 or more witnessed fits or if 1 fit lasts for more than 5 minutes: Rx Rectal diazepam (0.5mg/kg) or slow iv injection of diazepam (0.15mg/kg, maximum 10mg in an adult) Also correct hypoglycaemia if it is present.

10. Consider the need for blood transfusion: Look for signs of severe anaemia such as very pale mucous membranes, respiratory distress and a rapid pulse.
Note: The decision to transfuse with blood should not only be based on low laboratory values but as a guide Hct <15% or Hb<5 g/dL.

11. Exclude common infections/ conditions that present like severe malaria: Perform urinalysis for urinary tract infection; lumbar puncture for meningoencephalitis in unconscious patients (unless contraindicated); white blood cell count for other infections and chest x-ray for bronchopneumonia.

12. Observations & Appropriate Actions During Treatment:

i) Check level of consciousness:	If there is an altered level of consciousness use Glasgow or Blantyre coma scales to assess progress every 6 hours until fully conscious.
ii) Monitor Input/Output:	To detect dehydration and avoid fluid overload. Prevent pulmonary oedema by nursing the patient propped up at 45°.
iii) Ongoing monitoring of vital signs:	Measure vital signs every 6 hours to detect complications of severe malaria. If pulmonary oedema occurs (rapid respiratory rate and deep laboured breathing) stop all IV fluids, except quinine and call medical officer/clinical officer for assistance urgently.
v) Monitor parasitaemia:	Determine the parasite count daily to monitor the therapeutic effect of treatment. Stop when there is no detectable parasitaemia.
vi) Transfer to oral quinine:	Give tablets (crushed for an infant) when the patient can eat and drink.
vii) Counseling of patient/ attendant:	Health educate about compliance with a full course of treatment, home prevention of malaria and the sequelae of severe malaria. Wait for the patient to recover before counseling.

Produced by the Ministry of Health, in collaboration with the Malaria Consortium, with funding from Embassy of Ireland. Design by MeBK, Straight Talk Foundation.

Figure 4.3: Wallchart guidelines for management of the patient with severe malaria, Ministry of Health, Uganda

Below is a succinct description of the conditions associated with severe malaria and their management.

Anaemia

Anaemia is a common feature of *falciparum* malaria infection and may compound iron deficiency or nutritional anaemia. Severe malarial anaemia is predominantly found in children. Adults often develop mild anaemia which resolves when the parasitaemia has been cleared.

Management

Approaches used for management of anaemia are iron treatment and blood transfusion.

Iron treatment

Treat children with mild malaria and acute anaemia with iron. There is no evidence to show that iron treatment will worsen *falciparum* malaria. However, adding folate to anti-malarials appears to have no benefit. Folate may, in fact, interfere with the action of anti-malarials such as pyrimethamine-sulfonamide combinations.

Blood transfusion

Blood transfusion is normally only recommended for severe anaemia complicating *falciparum* malaria (see Table 4.2). This is because of shortages of blood and the risk of acquiring infections, such as HIV and hepatitis, through contaminated blood.

Timing of transfusion: The timing of blood transfusion is very important. In children with severe malaria anaemia, who have completed 48 hours of anti-malarial treatment, blood transfusion appears to offer little immediate benefit. Children with respiratory distress complicating severe malaria anaemia, however, need a blood transfusion as soon as possible, and even a delay of one or two hours can be fatal. A blood transfusion can act as a resuscitation fluid in children with respiratory distress characterised by acidosis, with little risk of pulmonary oedema developing.

Restricting blood transfusion: It has been suggested that blood transfusion should be restricted to children with severe anaemia who also have respiratory distress (see Chapter 3). Although this approach would prevent unnecessary transfusions, reduce the risk of blood-borne infection and conserve limited resources, it requires accurate identification of children with respiratory distress. It is also not known whether restricting transfusion to this extent is the best way of preventing unnecessary deaths. Therefore, where reliable, routine blood screening is carried out and blood supplies are adequate, a less restrictive approach to transfusion may be more appropriate.

Exchange transfusion: Exchange transfusion has been used in the treatment of *falciparum* hyperparasitaemia, particularly that associated with multi-organ dysfunction/impairment. However, this is a dangerous procedure, which must be carried out in an intensive care environment and there is no evidence to show that it prevents mortality.

Observe all patients with severe anaemia carefully. The development of respiratory distress should prompt immediate action. Infants are at greatest risk. Give blood more rapidly if the patient is shocked or is acidotic with poor peripheral perfusion.

If blood is being given to a patient who is well hydrated (normal blood and venous pressures and normal peripheral perfusion), you may use Frusemide (1 mg/kg up to 20 mg for an adult – rarely required in children, as they are often mildly to moderately dehydrated). It is not necessary if the patient is also dehydrated. Facilities for dialysis may be required if blood transfusion is thought necessary in a patient with established renal failure.

Table 4.2: Management of severe anaemia in malaria patients

Severe anaemia	
Adult	Haematocrit or Packed Cell Volume (PCV) < 20%
Child	Haematocrit or PCV 15%, Haemoglobin 5 g/dl
Treatment with blood transfusion	
	Packed cells 10–15 ml/kg over 4–6 hours or if not available use whole blood
	Whole blood 20 ml/kg over 4–6 hours (children may need as much as 30 ml/kg whole blood in cases of very severe anaemia)
Indications for blood transfusion	
Adult	Severe anaemia, if blood is readily available and if reliable infection screening can be performed
	Severe anaemia with respiratory shock that has not improved with intravenous fluid therapy and oxygen
Child	Severe anaemia with respiratory distress is an absolute indication for transfusion.
	Severe anaemia with hyperparasitaemia (> 20% red cells parasitized). Haematocrit or PCV < 15% or haemoglobin < 5g/dl

Convulsions

As noted in Chapter 3, convulsions (or fits) are more common in children than in adults. Convulsions in children which last longer than 30 minutes have been associated with a greatly increased risk of neurological sequelae.

Management

Treat convulsions lasting longer than five minutes with intravenous or rectal diazepam or with intramuscular or rectal paraldehyde. Intramuscular diazepam should *not* be given because it is not well absorbed. Treat prolonged convulsions aggressively, beginning with diazepam. Use paraldehyde if there is no response within five minutes after giving the right dose of diazepam. Give phenobarbitone or phenytoin if the child is still convulsing fifteen minutes after the first dose of diazepam.

If an individual has multiple convulsions (more than three in less than 24 hours), treat with a loading dose of phenobarbitone or phenytoin followed by maintenance doses until the resolution of the malaria.

You will also need to pay attention to the more general problems associated with convulsions:

- During the convulsion, turn the patient into the lateral position to avoid regurgitation and aspiration.
- Place a gag between the teeth to prevent biting the tongue. Take care not to insert your fingers into the patient's mouth.
- In the immediate period after the convulsion, use suction to maintain a clear airway. Do not forcibly attempt to control the airway *during* a convulsion: wait until the limb and body movements have stopped.
- If a convulsion lasts longer than five minutes, give humidified oxygen.

Coma

Some patients may spend many hours, even days in coma. Care of patients in coma should include the following:

- Nurse the patient in the lateral position to avoid regurgitation.
- If the patient is in deep coma and an impaired or absent gag reflex means there is a risk of aspiration, insert a nasogastric tube which can drain freely.
- Give fluids intravenously to maintain fluid balance in the patient.

Table 4.3: Anti-convulsants in severe malaria

Drug	Dosage and notes
Diazepam	0.2 to 0.3 mg/kg given IV for immediate control of convulsions. The dose may be repeated after 30 minutes up to a maximum cumulative dose of 1 mg/kg. 0.5 mg/kg given rectally for immediate control of convulsions Diazepam should not be given IM
Paraldehyde	0.1 ml/kg (using a glass syringe) by IV or IM injection for immediate control of convulsions 0.2 to 0.3 ml/kg diluted 1:1 with arachis oil give rectally for immediate control of convulsions
Phenobarbitone	15 mg/kg by IV infusion over 30–45 minutes for treatment of convulsions. Followed by 5 mg/kg (IM or oral) every 24 hours as a maintenance dose, if required
Phenytoin	15–18 mg/kg by IV infusion over 30–45 minutes for treatment of persistent convulsions. Followed by 5 mg/kg by IV infusion over 30 minutes every 24 hours, if required. Incompatible with dextrose solutions

- Aspirate unswallowed secretions from the oropharynx.
- Using one of the coma scales (see Table 3.3, page 56), monitor the depth of coma every six hours until the patient is conscious. A declining score is a bad sign; a persistent score may indicate the need for better treatment; an increasing score is an encouragement.
- Monitor vital signs such as temperature, respiratory rate, pulse, blood pressure and capillary refill time every six hours. In sophisticated settings, it is useful to monitor the blood gases and central venous pressure as well.
- Turn the patient every four hours to prevent pressure sores; bedding should always be kept dry because dampness increases the risk of pressure sores.
- Tape the eyelids closed to prevent damage to the patient's eyes.
- If the patient is in coma for more than 24 hours, give nutritional feeds down the nasogastric tube, according to daily nutritional requirements for his or her age. It is better to give small amounts frequently rather than filling up the stomach and increasing the risk of vomiting.
- Keep the patient clean by rubbing the body with a moist soft towel at least once a day. Dry with a soft towel.

Hypoglycaemia

Hypoglycaemia (blood glucose of ≤ 2.2 mmol/l) is often a complication of severe malaria in children and pregnant women. In Africa, at least 10% of children with severe malaria are hypoglycaemic on admission to hospital. The cause of hypoglycaemia may be different in adults and children, and there is less evidence in children of quinine causing hyperinsulinism than in adults.

Clinical diagnosis (see Chapter 3) is very difficult because the usual signs of hypoglycaemia are also found in malaria without complications of hypoglycaemia. But, since hypoglycaemia is associated with neurological problems and an increased risk of death, treat all pregnant women and children in coma for hypoglycaemia, if laboratory or bedside blood sugar measurements testing is not possible immediately.

Management

Treat acute hypoglycaemia with a slow bolus of intravenous glucose of 0.25-0.5 g/kg. This is equivalent to 0.5-1.0 ml/kg of a 50% glucose solution (which should be diluted in an equal volume of sterile water) or 2.5-5 ml/kg of a 10% glucose solution.

Give IV glucose over a period of five minutes. You *must* follow it immediately with a continuous infusion of glucose (see Shock, Step 4, below on maintenance fluids) to prevent rebound hypoglycaemia. Even children treated with a continuous infusion of glucose are at risk of further episodes of hypoglycaemia. Blood glucose should, therefore, be monitored every four hours until patients are conscious and able to take fluids orally. At this stage you can stop intravenous fluid therapy.

Shock

Shock is a serious sign. Classic 'warm' shock, sometimes observed in adults, may indicate co-existent septicaemia. Look for hypotension, tachycardia and acidosis which may be found with this type of shock, together with warm extremities and rapid capillary refilling. 'Cold' shock, which is more common in children in Africa, is characterised by hypotension, wide pulse pressure, tachycardia and acidosis, together with cool extremities and poor capillary refilling.

Management

1   In both warm and cold shock, the most important aspect of initial management, in addition to appropriate anti-malarial

treatment and possibly antibiotic therapy, is adequate fluid resuscitation. You can use the same management guidelines as for the treatment of dehydration. However, place greater emphasis on assessing:

- venous pressures and blood pressure in those with warm shock
- peripheral perfusion in those with cold shock
- urine output for quantity and colour in both.

2 The fluid you use in the resuscitation phase should be isotonic and contain physiological amounts of sodium (for example normal saline, Hartmann's solution or Ringer's lactate). You should not normally use solutions of dextrose, as they may cause hyponatraemia (low plasma sodium). However, if there is a risk of hypoglycaemia, give dextrose-containing fluids as maintenance fluids (see step 4 below) *in addition* to rehydration fluids. Urine output can only be usefully interpreted once a patient has been fully rehydrated (defined by normal blood pressure and venous pressures, good peripheral perfusion).

3 If urine output continues to be very poor (less than 0.5 ml/kg/hr in a child; less than 400 ml/day in an adult), diagnose renal failure and, if possible, transfer the patient to a more specialist unit. If this is not possible, then reduce fluid input to a minimum.

4 Once a patient is clinically rehydrated, give maintenance fluids intravenously if it is not safe or feasible to give fluids orally or nasogastrically.

- In children, use a solution of 4% dextrose/0.18% saline at 75 ml/kg/day (3 ml/kg/hr) for intravenous fluid maintenance. Add 10–15 mmol of potassium to each 500 ml bag of this fluid, unless there is persistent poor urine output (less than 0.5 ml/kg/hr).
- If 5% or even 10% dextrose are being used as maintenance fluids to treat or prevent hypoglycaemia, and it is expected that they will be used for more than six hours, then add 15–20 mmol of sodium and 10–15 mmol of potassium to each 500 ml bag of fluid.
- In an adult, 2–4 litres of fluid per day may be required for maintenance therapy, depending on the patient's size, temperature and urine output.
- If intravenous fluids are to be given for more than six hours, add sodium (30–40 mmol/l) and potassium (20–30 mmol/l) to avoid electrolyte imbalance. Stop intravenous fluids as soon as the patient is conscious and able to take fluids orally.

5 If a patient has been rehydrated adequately and poor urine output persists, indicating the presence of renal failure, you

should restrict intravenous fluid therapy. A standard regime of maintenance fluids may result in fluid overload in established renal failure. In this situation, give an amount of fluid intravenously that is equal to that passed out in the urine, with a small amount extra to replace fluid lost as sweat.

Although health workers have justifiable concerns about the development of pulmonary oedema, particularly in adults where it is a common cause of death, this should not prevent you rehydrating patients with severe malaria. In many cases, pulmonary oedema occurs without fluid overload where there is multi-organ impairment. Failure to correct dehydration can lead to established renal failure in adults and can prevent resolution of acidosis in children, with severe consequences.

Renal impairment

Diagnose renal impairment using careful assessment of a patient's state of hydration, to differentiate it from simple dehydration. Clinical signs are useful to identify dehydration, particularly in children. (See also Chapter 3.)

Most renal impairment in children can be reversed with adequate fluid management; in adults this is less clear. Specific management of established renal failure requires definitive support with dialysis – an intervention which is almost never available outside referral hospitals.

Management

If signs of dehydration are present, give boluses of intravenous fluid (10–20 ml/kg) over 30 minutes and then reassess the patient.

A moderately dehydrated child may require 40–50 ml/kg to complete rehydration. A more severely dehydrated child may require more fluid (manage as per diarrhoea/GE guidelines in IMCI manuals).

Adult reassessment should, if possible, include:

- clinical measurement of the jugular venous pressure (to check that it remains less than 2–3 cm above the sterno-clavicular angle with the patient seated at a 45° angle)
  OR

- measurement of central venous pressure (kept less than 5–6 cm of water when measured from the mid-thoracic point with the patient lying down).

Raised intracranial pressure

Several studies have found high intracranial pressure (ICP) in cerebral malaria with true coma (children with a Blantyre score ≤ 2, as opposed to a loose term for cerebral malaria that includes prostrated children).

Management

Even if ICP is high you may need to perform a lumbar puncture to help distinguish cerebral malaria and meningitis. Although lumbar puncture can have dangerous complications, the risk is difficult to quantify. One approach is to treat all individuals in coma for both meningitis and cerebral malaria initially, and to perform lumbar puncture when the patient is improving slightly or at least stable. Although culture of cerebrospinal fluid (CSF) after this time is unlikely to be useful, looking for the presence of a raised CSF white cell count more than 10 White Blood Cell (WBC)/ml) is still helpful in diagnosing meningitis.

There is currently little evidence to suggest that specific treatment to lower ICP is of any benefit, although anecdotal reports suggest it may be useful in some individuals. Specifically, steroids are not useful in severe malaria. Mannitol infusion is associated with a fall in ICP, but it is not known whether this translates to any improvement in outcomes.

High fever

High fever (hyperthermia) is especially common in children, and may contribute to convulsions and altered consciousness.

Management

Monitor rectal temperature frequently, and if it is above 39°C remove the patient's clothes, give tepid sponging and fanning, and administer paracetamol, 15mg/kg body weight by mouth, suppository or nasogastric tube.

Less common management issues

Pulmonary oedema

Pulmonary oedema carries a poor prognosis. Ideally, therapy should consist of mechanical ventilation and treatment of the underlying cause, for example dialysis to reduce volume overload in patients with renal failure. However, this may not be possible in many settings. You should use oxygen and diuretics, such as frusemide, to help manage the symptoms.

Bleeding

Although low platelet count (thrombocytopenia) is common in *falciparum* malaria, it rarely causes problems. However, severe bleeding problems, such as disseminated intravascular coagulation (DIC), do occur occasionally in adults. This needs supportive treatment using blood products in an intensive care environment.

Hyperparasitaemia

As discussed in Chapter 3, hyperparasitaemia is difficult to define, but it is usually treated in the same way as severe malaria, with the possible exception of a lower threshold for transfusion.

Assessment of recovery

Use records and observations, for example falling temperature, reduced parasite count and improved coma score to assess patient recovery. It is also important to assess the patient's ability to drink, eat, talk, walk, sit and stand.

When a patient has recovered, assess possible sequelae of the disease or of treatment by:

- performing a neurological examination to assess functional capacity to hold and use objects, ability to feed, and to do the things the patient was able to do before the illness. Assess language and memory
- assessing vision and hearing, using examination of the fundus oculi to assess retinal haemorrhage and simple bedside measures, especially for infants and children, such as whether the child turns its head towards a noise or watches the mother when she moves
- repeating haematocrit and blood films, ideally seven and fourteen days after recovery and again a month later. Reticulocyte response should be monitored. The haemoglobin (Hb) should not be continuing to fall on day seven. If it is, there may be another cause of the anaemia.

Case studies

4 *Jumoke has fits and is in coma*

Jumoke is three years old and had been unwell for three days when she presented to the health centre with a history of *recent fits*. At the health centre she fell from the chair she had been sitting on and had uncontrolled, rhythmic movements of her arms and legs, twitching of the mouth and rolling of the eyes, which lasted for five minutes. She had had a similar, shorter episode on the way to the health centre. She regained consciousness after the first fit, but 45 minutes after the second fit she was not responding to her mother's voice and was unable to sit up. The nurse advised the mother to take the child straight to the hospital, which was 20 minutes away.

At the hospital she was seen immediately by the doctor and examination confirmed that she had a *Blantyre coma score of 2*. She was also febrile, slightly pale, limp, had *reactive pupils and no obvious neck stiffness*. There was, however, some *intermittent but persistent slight twitching of the fingers of the right hand and the right corner of the mouth, and the eyes looked constantly to the left*. There was *no respiratory distress*; she had warm fingers and toes with *rapid capillary refilling* and only mild hepatosplenomegaly. A blood sample was sent for a parasite slide and measurement of haemoglobin and blood glucose (no other tests were available). Although she had no neck stiffness, a lumbar puncture was performed and this was found to be normal. When the blood film came back showing *falciparum* malaria, Jumoke was given IM quinine and IV maintenance fluids were prescribed.

Comment Jumoke's case is quite a typical story of severe malaria in African children, with coma appearing to begin after a convulsion. Such children must be treated quickly and correctly. In this case the nurse was right to make a rapid assessment and to refer Jumoke immediately rather than initiating treatment at the health centre. If, however, the journey to hospital had been longer, the nurse could have given, if available, IM quinine, IM artemether or artesunate suppository. The doctor was also correct in making a thorough assessment and not just concentrating on the obvious neurological problems. The decision to perform a lumbar puncture on admission is sometimes difficult (and depends on resources available), but it can provide valuable information. Knowing that the blood smear was positive for malaria does not exclude meningitis in malaria endemic areas where many asymptomatic children will also have a positive blood smear. The necessary parenteral treatment was started quickly. In this particular case, it might also have been beneficial to treat the child with an anti-convulsant such as diazepam. This is because very subtle seizures (the persistent twitching of the fingers and mouth with tonic eye deviation) may continue for very long periods, and treatment may result in rapid recovery from 'coma'.

5 Mtwali has breathing difficulty

Mtwali was *nine months old* when he presented to hospital with a two-day history of *fever* and *poor feeding* and a one-day history of *breathing difficulty*. On examination he was found to be very lethargic and *unable to breastfeed, very pale, with a rapid respiratory rate (60 bpm) and regular, deep breathing with nasal flaring*, and had mild hepatomegaly. He appeared to cry appropriately and watch his mother. It was not possible to measure Mtwali's blood pressure but his *capillary refilling time was prolonged at four seconds*. He had a PCV and a blood smear performed, and blood was sent to allow crossmatch for transfusion. These were the only investigations available, and showed a *PCV of 14%* and *falciparum* malaria on the blood film. He was admitted and prescribed intravenous quinine and a routine blood transfusion. Four hours later he deteriorated rapidly and became unconscious briefly, before having a cardio-respiratory arrest from which he died.

Comment   Respiratory distress, characterised by deep or acidotic breathing, is a medical emergency in a young child with malaria and severe anaemia. This boy also already had signs of poor peripheral perfusion on admission. He should have been given an urgent blood transfusion, ideally within 30 minutes of admission, which can correct hypovolaemia as well as anaemia. Frusemide is not indicated in such cases. An alternative explanation for the deterioration is hypoglycaemia, which should always be considered if there is a change in consciousness, and is treatable. Finally, diagnosing coma can be difficult in young children and in such cases careful observation of the child can provide important clues about the state of consciousness.

6 Unconscious Govinda

Govinda, a farmer, had been unwell with a *fever for about five days*. He had taken some medicines at home, but his relatives did not know which ones. Assessment at the local hospital found that he was conscious but *disorientated*, had no focal neurological signs, was mildly *hypotensive and had poor peripheral perfusion*. A blood film was taken and found to be positive for malaria. He was referred to the provincial hospital for further treatment, after starting on IV quinine for presumed severe malaria. Govinda was unconscious when he arrived at the provincial hospital four hours later, with a *Glasgow coma score of 7*. He was still *hypotensive, tachycardic, had poor peripheral perfusion and reduced skin turgor. His jugular venous pressure was undetectable* and he was mildly jaundiced. He was immediately given 500 ml of normal saline while investigations were carried out. These showed a normal blood sugar, haemoglobin of 9g/dl, normal electrolytes but an elevated plasma urea and creatinine. *An hour after the bolus of fluid, little had changed* and he had not passed urine.

Comment   This patient had been unwell for some days, had neurological impairment, hypotension and evidence of dehydration. A lumbar puncture could have been performed at the local hospital, or antibiotics could have been given until the possibility of meningitis had been excluded. Although he was started IV on an appropriate anti-malarial, he was not given any fluid resuscitation. Fluid resuscitation started several hours later, but there was already biochemical evidence of renal impairment. Prolonged hypovolaemia, secondary to dehydration, may also have contributed to the renal impairment.

This case illustrates the difficulty of deciding whether to give more fluids or whether to restrict fluid intake because of impending renal failure. The signs described suggest persistent dehydration, and the patient should therefore have continued to receive boluses of intravenous fluid (normal saline or equivalent) until his blood pressure and peripheral perfusion had improved. Fluid resuscitation should stop if the jugular or central venous pressure rises excessively.

Frusemide could have been given to address poor urine output at this point, but it should not be used before dehydration has been corrected. If urine output is still very poor (and a full bladder has been excluded) then renal failure should be assumed. Fluid intake should be restricted and renal function monitored regularly, with transfer to a unit capable of offering dialysis if possible. Once renal failure is present, drug doses need to be reduced.

Management of malaria at the periphery

An increasing number of countries are adopting the principles of Integrated Management of Childhood Illness (IMCI) and are developing country specific systems and protocols for implementing the system. *This system is designed specifically for use of primary level health workers at the periphery.*

Integrated Management of Childhood Illness

The Integrated Management of Childhood Illness approach has been developed by WHO and UNICEF. It combines improved management of childhood illness with aspects of nutrition, **immunisation** and other factors that contribute to child health. One of the key elements of the strategy is the training of first level health workers. A set of guidelines and training materials has been designed to give workers skills in the integrated management of the conditions that most frequently cause mortality in children in developing countries. The strategy is also intended to strengthen health systems. This includes the provision of **essential drugs,** the improvement of supervision and support of health facilities, strengthening of referral care and the reorganisation of work in health facilities. IMCI also helps to ensure appropriate action in the family and community to promote and sustain good childcare and to improve care-seeking for the child who becomes ill. IMCI provides a very useful model for the development of an effective, integrated approach to health care. It can be used by technical programmes, such as malaria control programmes, to achieve objectives in the area of child health.

The technical basis of the strategy is a clinical algorithm. In most countries it focuses on the five conditions that account, separately or together, for about 70% of childhood mortality (see Figure 4.4). The algorithm is designed to be adapted to the epidemiological and health service needs of each country, but in its generic form it covers:

- acute respiratory infections (ARI)
- diarrhoeal diseases
- fever, including malaria and measles
- ear infections
- malnutrition.

All children presenting with any illness are assessed for all of these conditions (in addition to any other illnesses they may present with that are not covered by the algorithm). IMCI gives guidance on the clinical management of children with these conditions as well as providing a base for preventive action and the

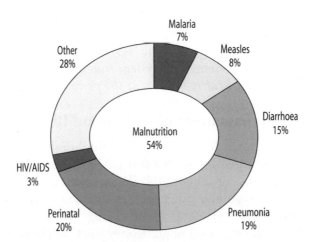

Figure 4.4: Distribution of 10.5 million deaths among children less than five years old in all developing countries, 1999

(Reproduced from *Model Chapter for Textbooks: Integrated Management of Childhood Illness 2001 www.who. int/mip.2001/files/2213/IMCI/ChapterApril01.pdf* by permission of WHO)

promotion of improved health. The nutritional status, including anaemia, of all children is also assessed.

The assessment process uses clinical skills only. It does not require laboratory facilities, and in most countries the only pieces of equipment used are a thermometer and a weighing scale.

The management of malaria in IMCI

How the algorithm works

Malaria is among the five most important causes of child mortality in a large number of developing countries, particularly in Africa. The generic IMCI algorithm was developed with this in mind, and the epidemiological status of malaria is used as a major determinant in the classification.

If you are assessing a child according to IMCI, you will need to follow this procedure.

Step 1: assessment for danger signs

Assess the child by checking for the three General Danger Signs: is the child able to drink or breastfeed; does the child vomit everything; has the child had convulsions? These are non-specific signs that the child is severely ill and in need of urgent attention, probably including referral. If the child has one or more danger signs but no other classification (see below), refer them urgently to hospital after a single dose of an appropriate antibiotic.

Step 2: assessment for main symptoms

After assessing for General Danger Signs, ask if the child has the following symptoms:

• a cough or difficult breathing
• diarrhoea
• fever
• an ear problem.

If the child has any of these symptoms, then the procedure is followed for the assessment and classification of that symptom. All main symptoms are covered in this way. By the time a child is assessed for fever, he or she will already have been assessed for General Danger Signs, cough or difficult breathing, and diarrhoea.

The procedure for all stages of classification, including the fever section is the same: identify signs by asking questions, looking and feeling. Use these signs to complete the right hand part of the table to classify the child (Figure 4.5). The classification blocks of the table are entered from the top in each case, the classification

MANAGEMENT OF THE SICK CHILD AGE 2 MONTHS UP TO 5 YEARS

Name: _____ Age: _____ Weight: _____ kg

Temperature: _____ °C

ASK: What are the child's problems? _____ Initial visit? _____

Follow-up visit? _____

ASSESS (Circle all signs present)   **CLASSIFY**

ASSESS	CLASSIFY

CHECK FOR GENERAL DANGER SIGNS
    NOT ABLE TO DRINK OR BREASTFEED
    VOMITS EVERYTHING
    CONVULSIONS
    LETHARGIC OR UNCONSCIOUS
	General danger signs present?
	Yes ____ No ____
	Remember to use danger signs when selecting classifications

DOES THE CHILD HAVE COUGH OR DIFFICULTY BREATHING?
• For how long? ____ Days
• Count the breathe in one minute.
      _____ breaths per minute.
      Fast breathing?
• Look for chest indrawing.
• Look and listen for stridor.	

DOES THE CHILD HAVE DIARRHOEA?
• For how long? ____ Days
• Is there blood in the stools?
• Look at the child's general condition. Is the child:
      Lethargic or unconscious?
      Restless or irritable?
• Look for sunken eyes.
• Offer the child fluid. Is the child:
      Not able to drink or drinking poorly?
      Drinking eagerly, thirsty?
• Pinch the skin of the abdomen. Does it go back:
      Very slowly (longer than 2 seconds)?
      Slowly?	

DOES THE CHILD HAVE FEVER? (by history/feels hot/temperature 37.5°C or above) Decide Malaria Risk: High Low • For how long? ___ Days • If more than 7 days, has fever been present every day? • Has the child had measles within the last three months? • Look or feel for stiff neck • Look for runny nose. Look for signs of MEASLES: • Generalised rash and • One of these: cough, runny nose or red eyes.	
If the child has measles now or within the last 3 months: • Look for mouth ulcers. If Yes, are they deep and extensive? • Look for pus draining from the eye. • Look for clouding of the cornea.	
DOES THE CHILD HAVE AN EAR PROBLEM?	

Figure 4.5: IMCI sample case recording form
(Permission is granted by the WHO to reproduce the IMCI sample case recording form from WHO/FCH/CAH/00.12 Annex B)

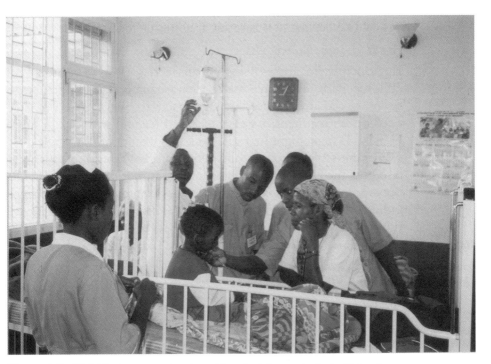

Figure 4.6: Child being examined and treated for malaria in Uganda

chosen being that which corresponds to the first box in the block in which positive signs are found. So, if a child has the sign of stiff neck, he or she would be classified as *very severe febrile disease* and you would look no further in that block. The child may, of course, at the same time have classifications in other blocks elsewhere in the algorithm. A child classified as *malaria*, for example, may also have signs requiring a classification of measles or dehydration.

Step 3: treatment

The treatment you provide will be determined by the classification. Details of the treatment to be given, adapted by each country as necessary, are given elsewhere in the IMCI guidelines.

The assessment of malaria in IMCI

The section of the IMCI algorithm that deals specifically with fever does not manage malaria on the basis of a specific diagnosis. The algorithm is actually for the management of fever generally. However, because malaria is the most important cause of fever-associated mortality, the local degree of intensity of its transmission is used as the basis for the major subdivisions.

The IMCI process is illustrated in Figure 4.7.

Areas of high malaria risk

In principle, in areas of high malaria risk (5% or more of all children with fever have malaria parasitaemia), all children with fever are classified as needing anti-malarials, whether or not they need other treatment as well. For a febrile child with one or more General Danger Signs or a stiff neck this would mean a single dose of intramuscular quinine followed by urgent referral. You would also give the child a dose of a suitable antibiotic and treatment to prevent hypoglycaemia. If the child has fever, but none of the signs indicating a need for referral, give oral anti-malarials and advise the mother to return in two days if the fever has not subsided or if the child's condition has become worse. The child may have other conditions that could cause the fever, but for safety's sake, treat this child for *both* malaria and the other condition(s).

Areas of lower malaria risk

Where the malaria risk is lower but still present, children are treated as having malaria in two circumstances. First, the classification of *very severe febrile disease* applies here also and needs to be treated as described above. Second, a child with fever, which apparently has no other cause, will be classified and treated as *malaria* following the national guidelines.

As can be seen in Figure 4.5 (page 116), the fever section includes the assessment of measles and its complications in all children who show signs of measles at the time of presentation or who have had measles in the past three months. Some countries have adapted the guidelines to include other locally important causes of fever, particularly dengue haemorrhagic fever.

WHO has prepared guidelines on managing children at first level referral hospitals, who have been referred from first level health facilities. These include standard recommendations on the management of the child with severe and complicated malaria.

Falciparum *malaria and pneumonia*

As noted above, the selection of signs for inclusion in the IMCI algorithm stresses the safety of the child. This is most obvious in the General Danger Signs, where no attempt is made to be specific as to the cause of the signs. The other significant non-specific sign in malaria endemic areas is fast breathing. This sign can be both sensitive and specific for respiratory infections requiring antibiotic treatment, except where there is a high incidence of malaria. The degree of crossover between *falciparum* malaria and pneumonia

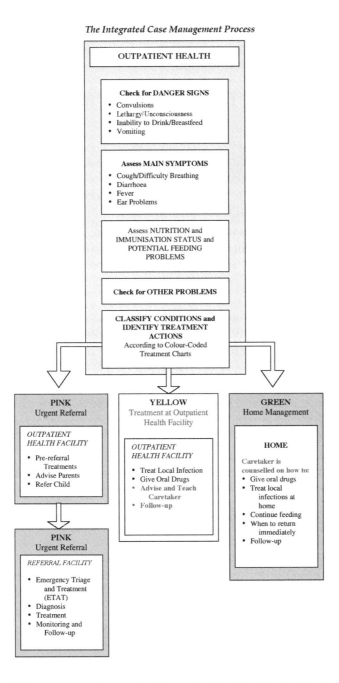

Figure 4.7: IMCI case management in the outpatient health facility, first-level referral facility and at home for the sick child from age two months up to five years (Figure reproduced from *Model Chapter for Textbooks: Integrated Management of Childhood Illness 2001 www.who.int/mip2001/files2213/IMCIChapterApril0.1pdf* by permission of the WHO)

in children with fever and fast breathing means that it is reasonable for the generic algorithm to recommend that such children be treated for both conditions.

The advantages of the IMCI strategy for malaria management

IMCI does not cover all malaria control activities. It does, however, offer a tool for strengthening the areas of a malaria control programme that focus on children.

The particular clinical advantage of the IMCI algorithm is that it treats each child for the full range of conditions. For example, a child with malaria will also be assessed for associated conditions such as anaemia. Mortality from all causes will be reduced if they are all detected and treated. At the same time it ensures that children with fever are detected and treated, even when fever is not the primary complaint.

IMCI promotes much wider involvement of health workers in the counselling of families on health protection and promotion. This could, where appropriate, include giving advice and support to families on, for example, the use of insecticide-treated mosquito nets.

The training component of the IMCI strategy brings together the training for a number of programme areas which are more usually separate. The broad and systematic programme of pre-service and in-service IMCI training offers malaria programmes an increased and more sustainable **coverage** of the training **target population**. This is equally true of other disease control programmes.

The introduction of IMCI by a country involves detailed adaptation of the IMCI guidelines and training materials. It is essential that these guidelines, which will be the basis for training and supervision of health workers at all levels, are fully in line with national guidelines. The IMCI guidelines also make recommendations on the selection and provision of drugs and equipment. Introduction of IMCI therefore provides an opportunity for the people responsible for malaria control in a particular country to review their own guidelines in conjunction with those who are providing other services to the same target population. This can lead to a clearer understanding between different disease programmes which have been working independently of each other, and offers the possibility of greater **efficiency** and effectiveness. For example, the combined voice of the concerned programmes can be particularly powerful in improving drug supplies.

The IMCI strategy stimulates efforts to rationalise and improve health care management in districts. It offers the advantages of more effective supervision and monitoring, greater efficiency of use of manpower, and improved referral of children with severe malaria and other serious conditions.

One of the dangers of the present extensive movement towards decentralisation in many countries is that it increases the risk of poor priority setting in decentralised systems and of fragmented health care. The inclusion of important parts of the malaria control effort in a clearly defined package with significant potential effectiveness makes it easier for decentralised managers to make appropriate choices.

Home care and management

Many people in malaria endemic countries obtain treatments for febrile illnesses from informal sources such as shops and kiosks. They will often only present for consultation at a health facility when this treatment in the informal sector fails. Self-medication is often more accessible and acceptable than seeking treatment at a health facility, but it is often not the correct treatment. Home care, however, is not always less correct than clinic care, and often has the advantage of being less expensive. Nevertheless, advice given at shops and the drugs themselves are both of variable quality. Shopkeepers and other sellers of drugs are untrained. Often the suppliers of over the counter (OTC) drugs are not aware of national treatment guidelines, and if they are, they do not use them.

Malaria home care programmes are being developed which aim to improve early home based treatment practices. Two main types of programme are used in different countries. One improves the practice of private providers (medicine sellers). The other recruits, trains and supports (with supplies and supervision) community-based drug distributors. The aim of the malaria home care programmes is to provide better access to, and information on, effective anti-malarial drugs for both users and providers. The challenge in the first type of programme is to facilitate quality treatment of malaria by an often unregulated and untrained, profit-oriented private sector.

There is increasing awareness that community or home-based treatment may be essential in efforts to reach all vulnerable people and to provide early effective malaria treatment. Critical steps in these programmes, which district health teams can support, include:

- engaging the community
- providing training or targeted communications for medicine shop owners or training for community drug distributors
- providing education and information to carers
- making effective prevention and treatment commodities widely accessible and affordable to families
- developing and using appropriate drug packaging/formulation
- influencing central political/regulatory activities.

Home care programmes have the potential to improve the effectiveness of treatment of the large proportion of malaria cases that do not reach public sector facilities. They can also build public-private partnerships to support facilities which are often under-staffed and under-resourced.

Management of severe malaria at the periphery

Most patients with severe malaria are seen at the primary health care level before they are referred or treated.

The priority for management of severe malaria is to recognise early on the clinical features that indicate severe malaria and the need for in-patient treatment. The symptoms and signs are non-specific (see Chapter 3).

The objective of management is to initiate treatment and to arrange referral as quickly and safely as possible. A patient with severe febrile disease may have severe malaria, meningitis or septicaemia. In most peripheral facilities, you will not have the laboratory facilities to distinguish which of these is the cause of the symptoms. The patient should therefore be urgently treated and referred.

If referral is not possible, then the treatment should continue with the patient kept at the health facility. However, clinical features that indicate that a patient *must* be referred, include:

- if still unconscious after 24 hours of quinine
- uncontrollable convulsions (for 30 minutes or more)
- severe pallor – these patients need an urgent blood transfusion
- renal failure
- pregnant women with severe malaria.

Delivery systems for case management

In addition to the choice of best drugs, the delivery system (this includes elements such as cost, availability, packaging of medication) has a great impact on its effectiveness. Broad health system policies can have a dramatic effect on access to treatment. For example, the introduction of user charges may deter people from using public sector facilities. On the other hand, the removal of user charges may lead to increased use, which in turn will reduce the availability of drugs.

Interventions using pre-packaged drugs (for example, in blister packs with dosage clearly indicated) have shown significant improvements in adherence to treatment regimens. In some instances, this may be partly due to greater patient education.

Poor access to treatment is a major but avoidable cause of illness and death. Different approaches have been made to bring adequate treatment closer to people at risk. One area of ongoing debate is which drugs should be available at what level of health service. Health workers in many first level facilities have successfully used drugs outside their normal authority, but parenteral treatment and use of second-line anti-malarials are often only considered appropriate at referral levels with trained staff. The use of artesunate suppositories has recently attracted much interest as a potential treatment of severe or potentially severe malaria, as they can be administered with less skill and fewer risks than injections. They are currently recommended as a starting dose for situations where IV or IM therapy is not possible, in particular prior to referral to a higher level health facility. Dosage is shown in Table 4.1 (page 100).

Delivery systems in the health unit that affect case management include the following:

1   Communication between staff – nurses, doctors and laboratory technicians, should be regular to facilitate teamwork.
2   Speed of diagnosis and commencement of treatment need to be emphasised.
3   Audits need to be done regularly to plan ahead to ensure that supplies/drugs meet demand on the wards.
4   Results of laboratory investigations should be communicated quickly and kept/recorded in an organised way for reference later on.
5   Case records should be properly stored and labelled so that they can be easily retrieved if the patient returns to the health facility.

Key points

> ▶ The most important principles of malaria case management are early and accurate diagnosis, prompt and effective treatment, adherence to treatment and provision of advice, follow-up and good nursing.
>
> ▶ Increasing drug resistance has led to adoption of artemisinin-based combination therapy (ACT) for treatment of *P. falciparum* malaria. As ACT is a recent introduction, extensive training is needed in its use and management. All health workers should have access to the latest national treatment guidelines.
>
> ▶ Regular monitoring of the efficacy of anti-malarials is essential using WHO standard protocols.
>
> ▶ Severe malaria must be treated as an emergency. Cerebral malaria and severe anaemia are the most common conditions associated with severe malaria. Delay in diagnosis and inappropriate treatment in infants and children are particularly dangerous.
>
> ▶ Access to prompt effective treatment may be enhanced for inaccessible vulnerable populations by supporting programmes to improve home care and management.

Further reading

1 WHO 1998a 'Planning for the implementation of IMCI in countries', WHO/CHS/CAH/98.1C
2 WHO 1998b 'Adaptation of the IMCI technical guidelines and training materials', WHO/CHS/CAH/98.1D
3 WHO 1998c 'IMCI training course for first-level health workers: Linking integrated care prevention', WHO/CHS/CAH/98.1E
4 WHO 1998d 'Follow-up after training: Reinforcing the IMCI skills of first-level health workers', WHO/CHS/CAH/98.1F
5 WHO 1998e 'The role of IMCI in improving family and community practices to support of child health and development', WHO/CHS/CAH/98.1G
6 WHO 2000a 'The Use of Anti-malarial Drugs. Report of a WHO Informal Consultation', WHO/CDS/RBM/2001.33
7 WHO 2000b *Management of severe malaria: a practical handbook*, second edition
8 WHO 2000c 'Severe and complicated malaria, third edition', Transactions of the Royal Society of Tropical Medicine and Hygiene, 94

9 WHO (2001) 'Anti-malarial Drug Combination Therapy', Report of a WHO Technical Consultation WHO/CDS/RBM/2001/35, reiterated in 2003 (Position of WHO's Roll Back Malaria Department on malaria treatment policy: *www.rbm.who.int/cmc_upload/0/000/016/998 who_apt_position.pdf*)

10 WHO (2003) 'Assessment and monitoring of anti-malarial drug efficacy for the treatment of uncomplicated *falciparum* malaria', WHO/HTM/RBM/2003.50 *www. who.int.malaria/docs/protocol-WHO.pdf*

11 WHO website reference for IMCI: *www.who.int/child-adolescent-heath/integr.htm*

12 WHO (2005) 'Susceptibility of *Plasmodium falciparum* to anti-malarial drugs: report on global monitoring: 1996–2004', WHO/HTM/MAL/2005.1103

Annex: Anti-malarial treatment schedules

(Adapted from 'The Use of Anti-malarial Drugs: Report of an informal consultation, 13–17 November, 2000. WHO/CDS/RBM/2001.33)

The first table (Table 4.4) shows a summary of indications, treatment schedules and contraindications for the major anti-malarials. Tables 4.5 to 4.12 provide detailed dosage schedules by weight and age.

Table 4.4

Drugs	When to use	Formulations	Frequency of dosage	Adverse effects	Contraindications
Artemisinin	In combination with blood schizonticides, for treatment of uncomplicated malaria Rectal administration for emergency treatment prior to referral in severe malaria, or in patients who cannot take oral medication.	1 Tablets and capsules containing 250 mg of artemisinin 2 Suppositories containing 100 mg, 200 mg, 300 mg, 400 mg or 500 mg of artemisinin	Monotherapy 20 mg/kg divided loading dose day 1, followed by 10 mg/kg once a day for 6 days Combination therapy 20 mg/kg divided loading dose day 1, followed by 10 mg/kg once a day for 2 more days + companion drug	Few adverse effects found in practice but may include headache, nausea, vomiting, abdominal pain, itching, abnormal bleeding and dark urine	Not recommended for use in the first trimester of pregnancy due to limited data on safety
Dihydro-artemisinin	In combination with blood schizonticides for treatment of uncomplicated malaria	1 Tablets containing 20 mg, 60 mg or 80 mg of dihydroartemisinin 2 Suppositories containing 80 mg of dihydroartemisinin	4 mg/kg in a divided loading dose in the first day, followed by 2 mg/kg daily for 6 days		

Drugs	When to use	Formulations	Frequency of dosage	Adverse effects	Contraindications
Artemether	In combination with blood schizonticides for treatment of uncomplicated malaria	1 Capsules containing 40 mg of artemether 2 Composite tablets containing 50 mg of artemether 3 Ampoules of injectable solution for intramuscular injection containing 80 mg in 1 ml, or 40 mg in 1 ml for paediatric use	Monotherapy 4 mg/kg loading dose on the first day, followed by 2 mg/kg once a day for 6 days Combination therapy 4 mg/kg once a day for 3 days, plus mefloquine (15 mg or 25 mg of base per kg) as a single dose or split dose on the second and/or third day Severe malaria 3.2 mg/kg by the intramuscular route as a loading dose on the first day, followed by 1.6 mg/kg daily for a minimum of 3 days or until the patient can take oral therapy to complete a 7-day course	No adverse effects have been reported in humans	Not recommended for use in the first trimester of pregnancy due to limited data on safety

Drugs	When to use	Formulations	Frequency of dosage	Adverse effects	Contraindications
Artesunate	In combination with blood schizonticides for treatment of uncomplicated malaria.	1 Tablets containing 50 mg or 200 mg of sodium artesunate 2 Ampoules for intramuscular or intravenous injection containing 60 mg of sodium artesunate in 1 ml of injectable solution 3 Suppositories of sodium artesunate	Uncomplicated malaria monotherapy 4 mg/kg loading dose on the first day, followed by 2 mg/kg once a day for 6 days Uncomplicated malaria combination therapy 4 mg/kg once a day for 3 days, plus mefloquine (15 mg or 25 mg of base per kg) as a single dose or split dose on the second and/or third day Severe malaria 2.4 mg/kg by the intramuscular route followed by 1.2 mg/kg at 12 and 24 hours, then 1.2 mg/kg daily for 6 days. If the patient is able to swallow, then the daily dose can be	No adverse effects have been reported in humans	Not recommended for use in the first trimester of pregnancy due to limited data on safety

Drugs	When to use	Formulations	Frequency of dosage	Adverse effects	Contraindications
			given orally. 2.4 mg/kg intravenously on the first day followed by 1.2 mg/kg daily until the patient can take artesunate or another effective anti-malarial orally Rectal administration see table x below		
Artemether-lumefantrine	Treatment of uncomplicated *P. falciparum* infections	Tablets containing 20 mg of artemether + 120 mg lumefantrine	In semi-immune patients 4-dose regimen consisting of 1, 2, 3 or 4 tablets taken at 0h, 8h, 24h and 48h. The total course for an adult is 16 tablets, which gives a total dose of 329 mg of artemether + 1,920 mg of lumefantrine	May cause dizziness and fatigue, anorexia, nausea, vomiting, abdominal pain, palpitations, **myalgia**, sleep disorders, arthralgia, headache and rash	Pregnant and lactating women Known hypersensitivity to either of the components Severe malaria

Drugs	When to use	Formulations	Frequency of dosage	Adverse effects	Contraindications
			Areas with multi-drug resistant P. falciparum and in non-immune patients Intensive 6-dose course is recommended, as in Table x below, at 0h and 8h, twice daily doses on the next 2 days is recommended. The course for an adult would be 4 tablets at 0h and 8h and 4 tablets twice a day on the 2nd and 3rd days		
Quinine	Treatment of severe P. falciparum malaria. 1st line in areas with multi-drug resistance IM for patients with uncomplicated malaria and constant vomiting 2nd line when resistance to	1 Tablets of quinine hydrochloride, quinine dihydrochloride or quinine sulphate containing 82%, 82% and 82.6% quinine base respectively Quinine bisulphate formulations,	Oral uncomplicated malaria 8 mg of base per kg three times daily for 7 days Where adherence may be a problem Quinine, 8 mg of base per kg three times daily for 3 days plus	Cinchonism in a high proportion of patients (ringing in the ears, high-tone hearing impairment, nausea and vomiting). May cause postural hypotension and hyperinsulinism, with the risk of hypoglycaemia An overdose may	

Drugs	When to use	Formulations	Frequency of dosage	Adverse effects	Contraindications
	1st line – should be used here in combination with another drug	containing 59.2% base are less widely available 2 Injectable solutions of quinine hydrochloride, quinine dihydrochloride or quinine sulphate containing 82%, 82% and 82.6% quinine base respectively	sulfadoxine 1500 mg or sulphalene 1500 mg plus pyrimethamine 75 mg given on the first day of quinine treatment Marked decrease in susceptibility of *P. falciparum* to quinine 8 mg of base per kg three times daily or 7 days *plus* doxycycline 100 mg of salt daily for 7 days (not in children under 8 years of age and not in pregnancy) or a loading dose of 200 mg of doxycycline followed by 100 mg daily for 6 days. *OR,* Tetracycline 250 mg 4 times daily for 7 days (not in children under 8 years and not in pregnancy) *OR,*	cause deafness and blindness as well as cardiac toxicity	

Drugs	When to use	Formulations	Frequency of dosage	Adverse effects	Contraindications
			Clindamycin 300 mg four times daily for 5 days (not contraindicated in children or in pregnancy)		
Chloroquine (CQ)	Uncomplicated chloroquine sensitive *P. falciparum* malaria *P. vivax, P. malariae* and *P. ovale* malaria	1 Tablets containing 100 mg or 150 mg of chloroquine base as a phosphate or sulphate 2 Syrup containing 50 mg of base as chloroquine phosphate or sulphate in 5 ml	Day 1: 10 mg/kg Day 2: 10 mg/kg Day 3: 5 mg/kg (see detailed schedule – table x below)	Itching common in dark skinned people Uncommon effects: nausea, mood or visual disturbances Very rarely, oral chloroquine can cause an acute and severe, but reversible, neuropsychiatric reaction IM or IV may cause hypotension and heart rhythm disturbances	Known hypersensitivity, epilepsy or psoriasis

Drugs	When to use	Formulations	Frequency of dosage	Adverse effects	Contraindications
Sulfadoxine – pyrimethamine (S-P)	Chloroquine resistant, S-P sensitive *P. falciparum*	1 Tablets containing 500 mg of sulfadoxine and 25 mg of pyrimethamine 2 Ampoules containing 500 mg of sulfadoxine and 25 mg of pyrimethamine in 2.5 ml of injectable	Single dose: 1500 mg of sulfadoxine and 75 mg pyrimethamine – comprises 3 tablets (see table x below)	Pyrimethamine: very safe, very rare may cause megaloblastic anaemia in those with folate deficiency Sulphonamide: severe skin reactions (rashes, blisters affecting the skin, mouth and eyes), hepatitis and blood disorders	Known **hypersensitivity**. In people with severe **hepatic** or renal dysfunction (except where the benefits exceed the risks involved) For **chemoprophylaxis** In infants < 2 months
Amodiaquine	In areas of resistance to chloroquine (though may be some cross resistance)	1 Tablets containing 200 mg of amodiaquine base as hydrochloride or 153.1 mg of base as chloro-hydrate 2 Suspension containing 10 mg of amodiaquine base as hydrochloride or chloro-hydrate	10 mg base per day for 3 days (see table x below)	Nausea, vomiting, abdominal pain, diarrhoea and itching. More rarely may cause toxic hepatitis and fatal **agranulocytosis** when used for chemoprophylaxis	Known hypersensitivity Hepatic disorders For chemoprophylaxis

Drugs	When to use	Formulations	Frequency of dosage	Adverse effects	Contraindications
Tetracycline	Can be used in combination with quinine in the treatment of *falciparum* malaria to decrease the risk of recrudescence It should not be used alone for treatment because of its slow action	Capsules and tablets containing 250 mg of tetracycline hydrochloride, equivalent to 231 mg of tetracycline base	High levels of resistance to quinine Quinine 8 mg of base per kg 3 times daily for 7 days + tetracycline 250 mg 4 times daily for 7 days Parasites are sensitive to quinine but adherence may be a problem Quinine 8 mg of base per kg 3 times daily for 3 days + tetracycline 250 mg 4 times daily for 5 days	May cause nausea, vomiting, diarrhoea and abdominal discomfort, transient depression of bone growth, discolouration of teeth, increased vulnerability to sunburn, rashes, itching Tetracycline should be kept out of the sunlight as in its degraded form it may cause renal dysfunction	Known hypersensitivity Pre-existing renal or hepatic dysfunction Children < 8 years and in pregnancy

Drugs	When to use	Formulations	Frequency of dosage	Adverse effects	Contraindications
Doxycycline	Can be used in combination with quinine in the treatment of *falciparum* malaria to decrease the risk of recrudescence It should not be used alone for treatment because of its slow action Chemoprophylaxis	Capsules and tablets containing 100 mg of doxycycline salt as hydrochloride	High levels of resistance to quinine Quinine 8 mg of base per kg 3 times daily for 7 days + doxycycline 100 mg of salt daily for 7 days *OR*, a loading dose of 200 mg of doxycycline followed by 100 mg daily for 6 days Parasites are sensitive to quinine but adherence may be a problem Quinine 8 mg base per kg 3 times daily for 3 days + doxycycline 100 mg of salt daily for 7 days *OR*, a loading dose of 200 mg of doxycycline followed by 100 mg daily for 6 days	May cause gastrointestinal irritation, increased susceptibility to sunburn transient depression of bone growth, and discolouration of teeth. Renal impairment may be aggravated but is less likely than with tetracycline	Known hypersensitivity Pre-existing renal or hepatic dysfunction Children < 8 years and in pregnancy

Drugs	When to use	Formulations	Frequency of dosage	Adverse effects	Contraindications
Mefloquine	Used for treatment of *P. falciparum* malaria only when known or suspected resistance to chloroquine and S-P Chemoprophylaxis	Tablets containing 274 mg of mefloquine hydrochloride, equivalent to 250 mg of mefloquine base	15 mg (in areas with no or low level resistance to mefloquine) or 25 mg (in areas of resistance to mefloquine) of mefloquine base per kg. (see table x below)	Nausea, vomiting, dizziness, weakness and mood disturbances quite common in adults With the exception of vomiting, these are less common in children. Mefloquine also exacerbates hypotension 1 in 1500 patients will experience temporary neuro-psychiatric reactions, such as convulsions or psychosis	History of allergy to mefloquine History of severe neuropsychiatric disease Those receiving treatment with halofantrine Those treated with mefloquine in the previous 4 weeks

Drugs	When to use	Formulations	Frequency of dosage	Adverse effects	Contraindications
Primaquine	Anti-relapse treatment in *P. vivax* and *P. ovale* infections Gametocytocidal drug in *P. falciparum* infections	Tablets containing 5.0 mg, 7.5 mg or 15.0 mg of primaquine base as diphosphate	Anti-relapse treatment in *P. vivax and P. ovale* infections In areas south of the equator where the Chesson strain of *P. vivax* is known to exist: 0.5 mg/kg for 14 days In areas north of the equator: 0.25 mg/kg for 14 days[2] Gametocytocidal drug in *P. falciparum* infections Single dose of 0.75 mg of base per kg base (adults; 45 mg of base); the same dose may be repeated one week later[3]	May cause nausea, dizziness and chest pain Most important is the risk of haemolysis in patients with G6PD deficiency.	Pregnancy. Children < 4 years Conditions predisposing to granulocytopaenia (reduction in the number of granulocytes – including neutrophils, basophils and eosinophils) including rheumatoid arthritis and lupus erythematosus

1 Where the patient is not able to be treated orally, the first dose of quinine should be given intravenously by slow infusion in isotonic fluid or 5% dextrose saline over 4 hours. If intravenous infusion is not possible, quinine may be given by intramuscular injection, the quinine should be diluted to a concentration of 60 mg/ml and divided into two halves, one delivered to each anterior thigh. Oral treatment should be resumed as soon as is possible.

2 G6PD deficiency should be excluded before standard doses of primaquine for anti-relapse are recommended. Use of primaquine in G6PD deficient patients may cause haemolysis.

3 Gametocytocidal treatment should only be given with or following schizonticidal treatment. It is not necessary to ascertain G6PD status as the dose given does not cause haemolysis.

Table 4.5: Dosage schedule for artemether/lumefantrine (Coartem®)

Weight (kg)	Age	No. of tablets (at 0, 8h, 24h, 36h, 48h and 60h)	Dose (Artemether/Lumefantrine)
5–14	<3 y	1	20 mg A + 120 mg L
15–24	3–9 y	2	40 mg A + 240 mg L
25–34	9–14 y	3	60 mg A + 360 mg L
≥ 35	>14 y	4	80 mg A + 480 mg L

Table 4.6: Dosage schedule for amodiaquine combined with oral artesunate for the treatment of CQ and S/P resistant resistant *P. falciparum* malaria

(Dose of amodiaquine 10mg/kg/day for 3 days; artesunate 4mg/kg/day for 3 days)

Weight (kg)	Age	Artesunate* 50 mg tabs	No. of amodiaquine tablets					
			# tabs of 153 mg base			# tabs of 200 mg base		
		# tabs	Day 1	Day 2	Day 3	Day 1	Day 2	Day 3
5–6	<4 m	$\frac{1}{2}$	$\frac{1}{2}$	$\frac{1}{2}$	$\frac{1}{4}$	$\frac{1}{2}$	$\frac{1}{4}$	$\frac{1}{4}$
7–10	4–11 m	1	1	$\frac{1}{2}$	$\frac{1}{2}$	$\frac{1}{2}$	$\frac{1}{2}$	$\frac{1}{2}$
11–14	1–2 y	1	1	1	1	1	$\frac{1}{2}$	$\frac{1}{2}$
15–18	3–4 y	2	$1\frac{1}{2}$	1	1	1	1	1
19–24	5–7 y	2	$1\frac{1}{2}$	$1\frac{1}{2}$	$1\frac{1}{2}$	$1\frac{1}{2}$	1	1
25–35	8–10 y	3	$2\frac{1}{2}$	$2\frac{1}{2}$	2	2	2	$1\frac{1}{2}$
36–50	11–13 y	4	3	3	3	3	2	2
50+	14+ y	4	4	4	3	3	3	3

* Artesunate is given daily for three days using the same daily dose

Table 4.7: Dosing schedule for mefloquine (250mg base) combined with oral artesunate for the treatment of multidrug resistant *P. falciparum* malaria
(Mefloquine: 25 mg/kg total; artesunate: 4 mg/kg/day)

Weight (kg)	Age	Day 1 Artesunate		Day 2 Mefloquine*	Day 2 Artesunate		Day 3 Mefloquine#	Day 3 Artesunate	
		# 50 mg tabs	# 200 mg tabs	# tabs	# 50 mg tabs	# 200 mg tabs	#tabs	# 50 mg tabs	# 200 mg tabs
5–6	3 m	$\frac{1}{2}$	$\frac{1}{4}$	$\frac{1}{4}$	$\frac{1}{2}$	$\frac{1}{4}$	$\frac{1}{4}$	$\frac{1}{2}$	$\frac{1}{4}$
7–8	4–7 m	1	$\frac{1}{2}$	$\frac{1}{2}$	1	$\frac{1}{2}$	$\frac{1}{4}$	1	$\frac{1}{2}$
9–12	8–23 m	1	$\frac{1}{2}$	$\frac{3}{4}$	1	$\frac{1}{2}$	$\frac{1}{2}$	1	$\frac{1}{2}$
13–16	2–3 y	2	$\frac{1}{2}$	1	2	$\frac{1}{2}$	$\frac{1}{2}$	2	$\frac{1}{2}$
17–24	4–7 y	2	$\frac{1}{2}$	$1\frac{1}{2}$	2	$\frac{1}{2}$	1	2	$\frac{1}{2}$
25–34	8–10 y	3	1	2	3	1	$1\frac{1}{2}$	3	1
36–50	11–13 y	4	1	3	4	1	2	4	1
51–59	14–15 y	5	1	$3\frac{1}{2}$	5	1	2	5	1
60+	15 y	5	1	4	5	1	2	5	1

* Vomiting is decreased if mefloquine is given on Day 2. If adherence is a problem, mefloquine dose can be given on Day 1.
# Mefloquine dose is 25 mg/kg, given as 15mg/kg on Day 2 followed by 10mg/kg on Day 3.

Table 4.8: Dosing schedule of sulfadoxine-pyrimethamine combined with oral artesunate for treatment of CQ resistant *P. falciparum* malaria
(Dose: 25 mg sulfadoxine/1.25 mg pyrimethamine/kg single dose; artesunate 4 mg/kg/day)

Weight (kg)	Age (years)	Day 1 SP*	Day 1 Artesunate		Day 2 Artesunate		Day 3 Artesunate	
		# tabs	# 50 mg tabs	# 200 mg tabs	# 50 mg tabs	# 200 mg tabs	# 50 mg tabs	# 200 mg tabs
4–10	< 1	$\frac{1}{2}$	1	$\frac{1}{4}$	1	$\frac{1}{4}$	1	$\frac{1}{4}$
> 10.1–14	1–2	$\frac{3}{4}$	1	$\frac{1}{4}$	1	$\frac{1}{4}$	1	$\frac{1}{4}$
> 14.1–20	3–5	1	2	$\frac{1}{2}$	2	$\frac{1}{2}$	2	$\frac{1}{2}$
> 20.1–30	6–8	$1\frac{1}{2}$	2	$\frac{1}{2}$	2	$\frac{1}{2}$	2	$\frac{1}{2}$
> 30.1–40	9–11	2	3	$1\frac{1}{2}$	3	$1\frac{1}{2}$	3	$1\frac{1}{2}$
> 40.1–50	12–13	$2\frac{1}{2}$	4	2	4	2	4	2
> 50	14+	3	4	2	4	2	4	2

* SP tablet contains 500mg of sulfadoxine and 25 mg of pyrimethamine

Table 4.9: Dosing schedules for SPas monotherapy (sulfadoxine-pyrimethamine, 500 mg/25 mg, Fansidar®, sulfalene-pyrimethamine 500 mg/25 mg)

(Use for the treatment of SP sensitive *P. falciparum* when artesunate is not available Dose: 25 mg sulfadoxine, sulfalene/1.25 mg pyrimethamine/kg single dose)

Weight (kg)	Age (years)	# tablets
4–10	< 1	$\frac{1}{2}$
10.1–14	1–2	$\frac{3}{4}$
14.1–20	3–5	1
20.1–30	6–8	$1\frac{1}{2}$
30.1–40	9–11	2
40.1–50	12–13	$2\frac{1}{2}$
> 50	14+	3

Table 4.10: Oral quinine regimens for the treatment of multi-drug resistant *falciparum* malaria

(10 mg salt/kg every 8 hours for 7 days)

200 mg tablet

Weight (kg)	Age	# 200 mg tablets	mg/kg dose received
< 8	< 8 m	$\frac{1}{4}$	7.1–10
8–12	7–24	$\frac{1}{2}$	8.3–12.5
13–17	2–4	$\frac{3}{4}$	8.8–11.5
18–25	5–8	1	8–11.1
26–35	9–11	$1\frac{1}{2}$	8.6–11.5
36–44	12–14	2	9.1–11.1
45–55	> 14	$2\frac{1}{2}$	9.1–11.1
≥ 55	> 14	3	8.6*–10.7

* for a 70 kg patient

300 mg tablet

Weight (kg)	Age	# 300 mg tablets	mg/kg dose received
7–11	6–14 m	$\frac{1}{4}$	6.8–10.7
12–23	15–6 y	$\frac{1}{2}$	6.5–12.5
24–37	7–12	1	8.3–12.5
38–52	13–> 14	$1\frac{1}{2}$	8.7–11.8
> 53	> 14	2	8.6*–11.3

* for a 70 kg patient

Table 4.11: Chloroquine dosage schedule using the 100 mg or 150 mg base tablets

(Use chloroquine alone only for the treatment of chloroquine sensitive *P. vivax*
Dose: 25 mg/kg chloroquine base total over 3 days)

Weight (kg)	Age (years)	Day 1	Day 2	Day 3	Day 1	Day 2	Day 3
		# 100 mg tabs			# 150 mg tabs		
5–6	< 4 m	$\frac{1}{2}$	$\frac{1}{2}$	$\frac{1}{2}$	$\frac{1}{2}$	$\frac{1}{4}$	$\frac{1}{4}$
7–10	4–11 m	1	1	$\frac{1}{2}$	$\frac{1}{2}$	$\frac{1}{2}$	$\frac{1}{2}$
11–14	1–2 y	$1\frac{1}{2}$	$1\frac{1}{2}$	$\frac{1}{2}$	1	1	$\frac{1}{2}$
15–18	3–4 y	2	2	$\frac{1}{2}$	1	1	1
19–24	5–7 y	$2\frac{1}{2}$	$2\frac{1}{2}$	1	$1\frac{1}{2}$	$1\frac{1}{2}$	1
25–35	8–10 y	$3\frac{1}{2}$	$3\frac{1}{2}$	2	$2\frac{1}{2}$	$2\frac{1}{2}$	1
36–50	11–13 y	5	5	$2\frac{1}{2}$	3	3	2
> 50	≥ 14 y	6	6	3	4	4	2

Table 4.12: Rectal administration of artesunate for emergency pre-referral treatment of severe malaria

Weight (kg)	Age (years)	Number of 100 mg capsules	Number of 400 mg capsules
10–19	1–5	1	–
20–29	6–7	2	–
30–39	8–12	3	–
40–49	> 12	–	1
50–90	> 12	–	2
> 90	> 12	–	3

5 ▶ The Prevention of Malaria

Chris Curtis and Jo Lines

This chapter describes:

▶ insecticidal control of adult mosquitoes

▶ larvicidal, biological and environmental control of mosquito larvae.

It discusses the implementation of preventive programmes through:

▶ mosquito net treatment

▶ house spraying

▶ larval control.

It will be useful for vector control supervisors, district health programme managers, as well as national policy makers and managers.

Introduction

Malaria can be prevented by controlling malaria mosquitoes, either by reducing the malaria mosquito population or by preventing them from biting. Although early diagnosis and prompt treatment are essential, they are not usually enough on their own to reduce malaria transmission. Mosquito control can be a highly effective and practical means of controlling malaria, both in endemic areas and during epidemics.

Mosquito (vector) control methods include those that:

- kill adult mosquitoes, and so reduce the survival rate of the adult mosquito population
- protect humans from mosquito bites
- reduce or prevent mosquito breeding.

The two most commonly used methods for killing adult mosquitoes include

- insecticide-treated mosquito nets (ITNs) and
- indoor residual spraying (IRS).

Methods that prevent mosquitoes biting humans include:

- ITNs
- untreated mosquito nets
- products for domestic use such as insecticide spays, coils, vaporising mats and repellents.

Methods that inhibit mosquito breeding include:

- environmental management to reduce breeding sources
- destruction of larvae through chemical or biological control.

Insecticidal control of adult mosquitoes

In rural areas, attacking adult mosquitoes with insecticide-treated mosquito nets (ITNs) and indoor residual spraying (IRS) is generally much more effective at reducing transmission than attacking mosquito larvae in the breeding sites. There are several reasons for this. One is that ITNs and IRS tend to reduce not only the number of vector mosquitoes, but also their survival rate. This is important because the malaria parasite takes ten days or more to

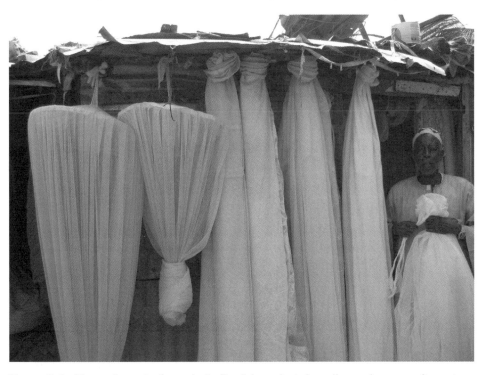

Figure 5.1: Mosquito nets for sale in Banjul market. Locally made mosquito nets are very popular in The Gambia.

mature inside the mosquito, and this is a long time in the life of the *Anopheles* mosquito. Even in the most favourable conditions, only a small minority of females live long enough to be able to transmit the parasite. In an area with many sprayed houses, or many treated nets, female mosquitoes risk being killed by the insecticide every time they enter a house to seek a meal, which they do every two or three days. In this way, ITNs and IRS can greatly reduce the proportion of vectors that live long enough for the malaria parasite to mature inside them. This in turn greatly reduces the capacity of the local vector population to transmit malaria.

These methods of attacking adult mosquitoes also have the advantage of being relatively standard in their technical requirements. A house-spraying operation in one region involves much the same activities, resources and skills as in another. Attacks on breeding sites, on the other hand, require considerably more adaptation to local conditions, because the breeding sites that are important vary greatly from place to place and from species to species.

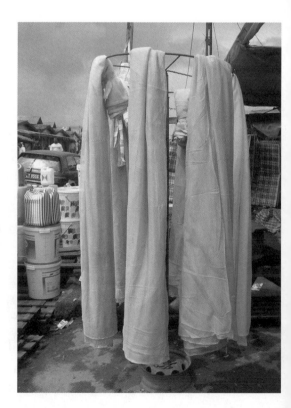

Figure 5.2: Nets in Douala market, Cameroon. In some countries nets are sold together with insecticide for home treatments.

Insecticide-treated mosquito nets (ITNs)

As most *Anopheles* mosquitoes bite late at night when people are sleeping, mosquito nets hung over the sleeping place can provide an effective physical barrier. However, mosquitoes will still bite people if there is a small hole or tear in the net, or if any part of the body is touching the net. Treating a net with insecticide can make it a much more effective barrier. A net dipped in a pyrethroid insecticide can kill or repel mosquitoes so that they do not try to enter the net, or to bite the person through the net. **Pyrethroids** on nets are safe for adults and children, including babies who may suck a treated net.

Distribution and delivery of ITNs

ITN projects have been implemented in many countries since the 1980s. Since the launch of RBM (Roll Back Malaria) in 1998, there has been increasing recognition of the need to scale up from small projects to large programmes that achieve national coverage. The best way of achieving large-scale coverage and overcoming the challenges of '**going to scale**' is through the development of a national co-ordinated programme. The role of the district is to support the implementation of the national ITN strategies that this programme develops.

The capacity of the public sector to provide ITNs for everyone, and to sustain this provision, depends on the size of the population, on the resources available and other competing demands on these resources. Capacity will vary from country to country. It is, however, more likely to be adequate in places where malaria is localised than in those where most of the population is at risk. In recognition of the difficulties faced by ITN programmes in countries where most of the population is at risk, the RBM Technical Support Network on ITNs developed the '*Strategic framework for co-ordinated national action: Scaling up insecticide-treated netting programmes in Africa*'. This document proposes strategies for scaling up ITN use that are effective, affordable and sustainable in the long term. These combine sustained public provision of targeted subsidies, aimed at maximising public health benefits, with stimulation and support of the private sector.

Districts need to ensure that their strategies and those of their partners, i.e. NGOs and community-based organisations (CBOs), fit with those of the national level in terms of:

- the use of subsidies
- the anticipated role of and relationship with the private sector

- definitions of the target group for receipt of the subsidy
- mechanisms of targeting.

There is general agreement that high ITN coverage is desirable and that this will require use of substantial and sustained subsidies. Some argue that subsidies should be targeted to the most vulnerable groups, such as pregnant women and children, or to the poorest.

Information, education and communication (IEC)

Any system for increasing the use of ITNs needs a good IEC component both to ensure demand and correct use (when and how to use, who should use, when and how to retreat).

Treating mosquito nets with insecticide

Treating mosquito nets with insecticide is a simple procedure, but technical and safety guidelines need to be followed. The net is immersed in the insecticide mixture in a bowl or a plastic bag, soaked and kneaded thoroughly, wrung out and laid out to dry.

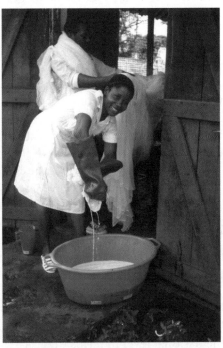

Figure 5.3: Annual treatment of a mosquito net with pyrethroid insecticide

The amount of water needed depends on the material of the net. Cotton nets absorb much more liquid per square metre than synthetic nets, such as polyester or nylon. Standard recommendations are:

- 0.5 litre of water for one medium-sized synthetic net
- 2 litres of water for one medium-sized cotton net.

However, if the net is very large or very thick, extra water may be needed. So, after working out the amount of insecticide to use (see Table 5.1), you need to work out the amount of water. You will need enough water to wet the whole net thoroughly, but not so much that a lot of the insecticide solution will be left behind, or will drip out. Measure this by dipping a net in water. You can measure the volume absorbed either directly, with a measuring cylinder, or by weighing the net dry and then wet (1 ml of water weighs 1 gm).

Table 5.1 lists the insecticides recommended for net treatment by the WHO Pesticide Evaluation Scheme (WHOPES), and the doses required to kill mosquitoes that land on them. Generally a net can be washed several times and the insecticide will still be effective. However, repeated washing does gradually remove the insecticide, so the nets must be retreated annually.

Important note: Check the concentration of the insecticide on the label of the container. Concentrations listed in column one of Table 5.1 are percentages. Some manufacturers list concentrations as gm/litre.

If concentrations are presented as gm/litre divide by 10 to obtain the % concentration, for example 25 gm/litre = 2.5%

If you are treating more than one net, multiply the insecticide and number of litres of water by the number of nets to be treated. For example, treatment of three synthetic nets with 5% Cyfluthrin would require 3 × 15 ml of insecticide in 3 × 0.5 = 1.5 litre of water.

When you are dipping nets made of the same material, but of different sizes in the same bulk insecticide solution in a bowl, you do not need to measure the area of each net. This is because each net will absorb liquid in proportion to its area. However, if you are treating the nets individually, it is important to assess the size of each net to estimate the volume of liquid required.

Table 5.1: Pyrethroids and related insecticides used for treatment of mosquito nets

Chemical	Trade names	Formulation	Target dose	Amount of concentrate for one medium size net (15 m²)	Amount of concentrate to be added to 10 litres of water to treat 20 synthetic nets	Amount of concentrate to be added to 10 litres of water to treat 5 cotton nets*
Permethrin 10%	Imperator/ Peripel	EC	200–500 mg/m²	75 ml	1,500 ml	375 ml
Deltamethrin 1%	K-othrin	SC	15–25 mg/m²	40 ml	800 ml	200 ml
Deltamethrin 25%	K-Otab	WT	15–25 mg/m²	1 tablet (1.6 g)	20 tablets	5 tablets
Lambda-cyhalothrin 2.5%	Icon	CS	10–20 mg/m²	10 ml	200 ml	50 ml
Cyfluthrin 5%	Solfac	EW	50 mg/m²	15 ml	300 ml	75 ml
Etofenprox 10%†	Vectron	EC/EW	200–500 mg/m²	30 ml	600 ml	150 ml
Alpha-cypermethrin 10%	Fendona	SC	20–40 mg/m²	6 ml	120 ml	30 ml

(Adapted from: *Instructions for treatment and use of insecticide-treated mosquito nets:* WHO. WHO/CDS/RBM/2002.41 WHO/CDS/WHOPES/GCDPP/2002.4)

NOTE: formulations abbreviated as follows:
EC = emulsifiable concentrate
SC = suspension concentrate
CS = microencapsulated
WT = wettable tablet
EW = oil-in-water emulsion
* cotton nets absorb much more water than synthetic nets
† this is not a pyrethroid

Safety guidelines

Pyrethroids are safe for humans, particularly in the doses used for treating nets and curtains. However, when handling concentrated insecticide or carrying out mass retreatment of many nets (i.e. if you are dipping nets all day), you are strongly advised to wear protective clothing: masks, safety glasses, elbow-length gloves, overalls and preferably rubber boots Where large bowls of insecticide solution are to be used for communal dipping, you may wish to wear safety glasses to avoid splashes in the eye.

Always dispose of surplus solution safely, for example in a pit latrine or buried in dry ground away from buildings, where it will rapidly become harmless. Never pour it into small rivers or streams, or on land where it could drain into these. Although pyrethroid insecticides are relatively safe for humans, they are very toxic to fish. Destroy empty insecticide containers or clean them very carefully to avoid the risk of using contaminated containers for food storage.

Checking the insecticidal power of the net

Exposing mosquitoes to treated netting can easily be done to check, or to show community members, either that an adequate insecticide dose has been achieved on nets or that retreatment is necessary. One project did this by creating a 'bag' of treated netting which is wrapped tightly around a wire frame. Live *Anopheles* mosquitoes are collected from houses with no treated nets and placed inside the bag. The time for each mosquito to be killed by the insecticide is measured, using the second hand of a watch. With a good insecticidal deposit, this should be less than ten minutes. The time taken will increase when the net has been repeatedly washed, and decrease after it has been retreated.

Insecticide retreatment

Nets should be retreated annually, or twice a year, if recommended. Strategies for retreatment should emphasise the treatment of *all* mosquito nets – including locally made nets that have not previously been treated. A retreatment programme needs to aim for high community coverage in order that the maximum number of mosquitoes are killed.

Nets can be treated and retreated either individually or in large batches. You need to determine which of these methods is the more appropriate, depending on the preferences of your community and the resources you have available. Delivery mechanisms for retreatment include:

- mass treatment campaigns which can provide quick and comprehensive coverage for almost all nets in a community
- fixed treatment services, where people are able to take their nets when they wish
- mobile treatment services, which may involve market days or door-to-door agents
- dip-it-yourself treatment kits, for individual net treatment that people can use in their own home.

In some places, dip-it-yourself sachets come with illustrated leaflets in the local language. These provide detailed information for home use; for example, how to measure the correct volume of solution for common sizes of nets, using a locally available container such as a soft drink bottle.

Long-lasting insecticidal nets (LLINs)

Nets are now being manufactured in which a pyrethroid insecticide has been incorporated into the plastic even before it is made into fibre, or in which the pyrethroid is applied to netting in the factory in combination with an adhesive resin. Good-quality versions of these long-lasting insecticidal nets (LLINs) remain insecticidal for longer and after more washes than is the case with conventionally dipped nets. It is claimed that LLINs will remain insecticidal for the whole physical 'life' of the net.

LLINs are, at present, more expensive than conventional nets, but the widespread use of LLINs would avoid the need to organise and pay for net retreatment.

Insecticide-treated curtains

In areas where vector mosquitoes bite at times when people are not sleeping, insecticide-treated curtains over openings such as windows, doors and eave gaps may sometimes be preferable to mosquito nets. These can be very cheap, especially where openings are small. Possible disadvantages of insecticide-treated curtains compared with mosquito nets include: people may prefer to have a mosquito net, curtains are more difficult to take down to retreat, and door curtains are often not kept in place.

Indoor residual spraying (IRS)

A successful but more demanding method of preventing malaria is indoor residual spraying. An insecticide is sprayed on to the inside walls and ceilings (or the underside of the roof if there is no ceiling) to kill female *Anopheles* mosquitoes when they come indoors to bite. The type of insecticide used is one that sticks to the surface and will continue for some months to kill insects that land on the surface. This is different from aerosol sprays that kill mosquitoes in the room at the time of spraying, but which do not last.

Experience has shown that, even in settings where malaria eradication is not a realistic objective, an effective spraying programme that covers most houses in a community can greatly reduce the burden of malaria. In some cases, effective house spraying has, at least temporarily, eradicated some of the more easily killed malaria-transmitting mosquito species, such as *Anopheles funestus* in parts of Africa.

Mosquitoes which rest indoors

Most, but not all, of the mosquitoes that pose the greatest danger of transmitting malaria rest indoors before and/or after biting. This is because:

- malaria mosquitoes tend to bite when people are asleep and usually have to come indoors to find sleeping people.
- *A. gambiae* and *A. arabiensis* in Africa have their main biting times between 10 pm and 4 am.
- mosquitoes find it difficult to fly far with a blood meal inside them, as it approximately doubles their weight – most species are likely to remain in the room after biting.
- in hot dry countries, houses are relatively humid and cool places for mosquitoes to spend the day.
- some mosquitoes which bite cattle outside come indoors to rest.

Box 5.1: House-spraying conditions

Four conditions are essential for the success of house-spraying programmes:

▶ Coverage: the proportion of houses and rooms in the community sprayed is high enough (greater than 80%) to ensure that few mosquitoes escape.

▶ The malaria mosquitoes in the area belong to a species which enters and rests inside houses for long enough to pick up insecticide placed there.

▶ The mosquitoes are susceptible to the insecticide being used.

▶ The insecticide is applied safely and the community has confidence that this is so. It also helps if they observe the beneficial side effects of the insecticide in eliminating other domestic nuisance insects.

Species of mosquitoes which come indoors to rest and are suitable for attack by house spraying include: *A. gambiae* and *A. funestus* in tropical and southern Africa; *A. darlingi* in northeastern South America, and *A. culicifacies* and *A. fluviatilis* in the Indian sub-continent. *A. albimanus* in Central America and northwestern South America is less likely to rest in the house. In Southeast Asia, *A. dirus* leaves houses immediately after blood feeding, while *A. minimus* has changed its behaviour since house spraying was introduced and in many areas no longer rests in houses.

Before starting or restarting a spraying programme, the first step is to find out about malaria mosquito habits. If you do not know for certain whether malaria mosquitoes rest indoors, it is advisable to check. This is done by collecting mosquitoes resting inside houses early in the morning, using an electric torch and entomologists' sucking tubes or test tubes. The collected mosquitoes should be inspected to see if they include *Anopheles*. (See Chapter 1: The Biology of Malaria, page 13, on how to distinguish *Anopheles* from other mosquitoes.) If you find that there are *Anopheles* females resting in houses, the next step is to identify the species, consider what insecticides are available and whether the local *Anopheles* species is susceptible to them.

Selecting an insecticide for house spraying

Mosquito susceptibility and resistance

The insecticides most commonly used for house spraying are listed in Table 5.2. Initially, all *Anopheles* were susceptible to these insecticides, but resistance has now evolved in some mosquito populations. Resistance to an insecticide (or, in certain cases,

Table 5.2. Insecticides commonly used for house spraying against malaria mosquitoes (partly based on Rozendaal, WHO, 1997)

Chemical	Class	Trade name	Dose (gm a.i./sq m)	Persistence (months)	Toxicity problems
DDT	OC	–	1–2	6 or more	Residues in breast milk
Malathion	OP	–	2	2–3	Odour; can be contaminated
Fenitrothion	OP	Sumithion	2	3–6	Attacks cholinesterase
Pirimiphos-methyl	OP	Actellic	1–2	2–3	None known
Bendiocarb	Carb.	Ficam	0.1–0.4	2–6	Toxic but available in sachets
Deltamethrin	Pyr.	K-Othrin	0.01–0.025	2–3	Irritant
Lambda-cyhalothrin	Pyr.	Icon	0.02–0.03	3–6	Irritant

Note: insecticide classes abbreviated as follows:
OC = **organochlorine**
OP = organophosphate
Carb. = carbamate
Pyr. = pyrethroid
a.i. = active ingredient

cross-resistance to several different insecticides) is due to an inherited mutant gene or genes. Spraying with a particular insecticide will kill most of the mosquitoes that do not have the mutant gene or genes. This means that the proportion of mosquitoes that survive with the mutation, the breeding population, will increase towards 100%, through a process of evolution.

To find out whether the local malaria mosquito population has developed resistance to a particular insecticide, expose a sample of mosquitoes to a dose of insecticide which will normally kill susceptible mosquitoes. (Papers treated with doses of the insecticides listed in Table 5.2, and test kits of plastic tubes, are available from WHO via University of Penang, Malaysia, through in-country WHO offices or on the WHO malaria website.) Mosquitoes should be kept in contact with the treated paper for one hour and then held in a tube with untreated paper for 24 hours, during which time delayed effects of the insecticide may occur. If 100% of the mosquitoes are killed, there is full susceptibility and if 100% survive there is complete resistance.

If the kill is less than 80% you should use a different insecticide. The insecticide you choose should be the most effective available one that you can afford. Changing the insecticide may be a complicated process and there are likely to be delays between ordering and delivery. The existence of even a low percentage of mosquitoes with a resistance gene means that the process of evolution has already begun and will probably evolve further in the presence of an extended spraying programme.

Safety considerations

Another important consideration in the choice of insecticide is safety to humans, domestic animals and wildlife. All the insecticides listed in Table 5.2 are approved by WHO toxicologists as safe for house spraying, provided that appropriate precautions are taken.

Organochlorines (DDT)

DDT (dichlorodiphenyltrichloroethane) has acquired a very bad reputation because its heavy use against agricultural pests has resulted in harmful accumulations of the insecticide in wild birds and fish. The Stockholm Convention on Persistent Organic Pollutants, which was signed in 2001, contains an amendment which authorises the use of DDT specifically for vector control. WHO has continued to recommend its use for household spraying against malaria mosquitoes, provided that the mosquito population concerned is not resistant to it.

In many Latin American and Asian countries, DDT is being, or has been, phased out from anti-malaria use because it is perceived to be environmentally harmful. This can cause problems in areas where all the alternatives are considered to be too expensive, so house spraying stops. For example, there is evidence from Latin America that the phasing out of DDT has coincided with a resurgence of malaria. In South Africa and Madagascar DDT was phased out, but there has since been successful reversion to DDT spraying. Fears in the past that DDT was associated with cancer were not backed up by evidence. There remains some doubt regarding reported associations with developmental outcomes and/or potential endocrine effects, but these associations have not been shown to be causal, and there is currently no conclusive nor convincing evidence that DDT is harmful to human health in any way.

Organophosphates and carbamates

Organophosphates and **carbamates**, such as **malathion, fenitrothion** and **bendiocarb**, are used at approximately the same dose as DDT, but the cost per house sprayed is much higher.

- Malathion of good quality is relatively safe, although contaminated batches have caused harm to sprayers in the past, so assurance about quality control is important. Even good quality malathion smells unpleasant when sprayed and its durability on mud surfaces is poor.
- Fenitrothion is an organophosphate, like malathion, but is effective against some mosquito populations which are resistant to malathion. Where fenitrothion is being used, sprayers should be checked for the level of cholinesterase in their blood. A simple test kit for this can be obtained from in-country WHO offices. Any individuals showing more than a 25% reduction from their initial level of cholinesterase, should be taken off spraying duties until the level returns to normal.
- Bendiocarb is a relatively toxic insecticide, but it is available in soluble sachets of a size sufficient for one-spray pump filling. This avoids skin contact with the insecticide powder, which poses the greatest risk of harmful absorption to sprayers.

Pyrethroids

Many countries are switching to pyrethroids, such as **deltamethrin** or **lambdacyhalothrin**, for malaria mosquito control. Although they seem more expensive, pyrethroids can be used at far lower doses than other classes of insecticide, and this should be taken into account when comparing prices. Pyrethroids are considered to be the safest class of insecticide, but they can cause sneezing or unpleasant irritation to the skin during spraying operations, so careful handling, protective clothing and face visors are as important as they are with other insecticides.

Safe application

During spraying operations, sprayers should wear:

- overalls
- a cap or hat with a broad peak or brim to minimise insecticide droplets falling on to the face
- good quality rubber gloves
- rubber boots.

If possible, and especially if more irritant insecticides such as pyrethroids are being used, sprayers should wear goggles and gauze face masks or plastic visors to completely screen the face. Sprayers should not take overalls and other protective clothing home. Protective clothing must be washed regularly.

Make sure that soap and water are easily available so that sprayers can wash their hands and faces during and at the end of the working day. It is important that the spray team leader knows where to obtain medical help in the event of organophosphate or carbamate poisoning. Make sure that the antidote, atropine (2–4 mg for adults), is available for injection (Rozendaal, WHO, 1997).

Householders need advance warning that a spray team is coming. Ask them to make sure that children, domestic animals, food, cooking utensils, clothes and small items of furniture are not in the house during spraying and for half an hour after spraying has been completed. Where large stores of food, such as maize cobs, are stored inside houses, it may not be feasible to remove them and, instead, they should be carefully covered with impermeable plastic sheets before spraying.

The spray team supervisor plays an important role, especially in making contact with householders and ensuring they understand that the spraying is being done to protect their families against malaria mosquitoes. The supervisor also needs to explain that it will only be successful if all rooms, especially the bedrooms, are sprayed. He or she should check that children, animals and the items mentioned above have been removed from the house before spraying, and keep a record of how many and what proportion of rooms were sprayed.

After spraying, empty insecticide containers should be destroyed or carefully cleaned, to avoid the risk of contaminated containers being used for food storage. Arrange for residues from spray pumps to be tipped down pit latrines or buried in dry ground away from houses and children. Pump contents must not be emptied where they can drain into water courses, because many insecticides are much more toxic to fish than they are to mammals.

Implementing house spraying

A compression sprayer (see Figure 5.4), such as a Hudson X-pert, is used for house spraying. After introducing the insecticide suspension, the pressure in the tank is pumped up by hand to 2.8 kg/sq cm. Operation of the trigger releases the flow through the nozzle. As the tank is emptied:

- the pressure gauge should be checked and the pressure pumped back up to 2.8 to ensure a standard flow rate. (Some modern machines come with pressure regulators which ensure a standard flow rate within a wide pressure range in the tank.)
- the flow rate should be periodically checked with a measuring cylinder and the second hand of a watch. The rate should be 750 ml/minute.

Serious deviation from the correct flow rate is usually due either to the nozzle being partially blocked or being worn, so that the opening has become too wide. Make sure that spare nozzles, rubber washers and gaskets are available and that the spray team includes someone with sufficient mechanical skills to fit spares and carry out simple repairs. At the end of each working day, spray pumps must be thoroughly cleaned and left to drain dry.

The pump nozzle can also be damaged by sand grains in well water. To remove the sand, filter the suspension or the water being poured into the pump through coarse cloth (the insecticide powder is so fine that it will pass through this).

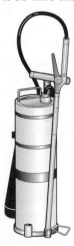

Figure 5.4: The Hudson X-pert compression sprayer
(Source: *www.hdhudson.com*)

Insecticide is sprayed indoors and under the eaves outdoors (see Figure 5.5). In use, the nozzle is held 40 cm from the wall, ceiling or roof. A long lance will be needed for high roofs. The correct type of nozzle emits an 80° fan of insecticide spray and the lance is held so that the fan is in the horizontal plane. The lance should be swept steadily up and down to create slightly overlapping vertical swathes of sprayed surface. Spraying should be done at a speed that applies 50ml/m². This amount will wet most types of wall surface evenly without run-off. With an emission rate of 750 ml/minute the aim is to cover 750/50 = 15 m²/minute.

Table 5.2 (page 152) indicates the length of time (in months) that insecticide deposit on a wall should remain effective. Where malaria is seasonal, however, it may only be necessary to spray just before the beginning of each malaria season.

Spray teams can be trained, using a wall with vertical lines marked 50 cm apart and two metres high, to spray fifteen of these 1 m² strips in a minute. Once they can do this on a straight wall, training should continue in the more confined and difficult conditions of small houses where walls, ceilings and roofs have to be

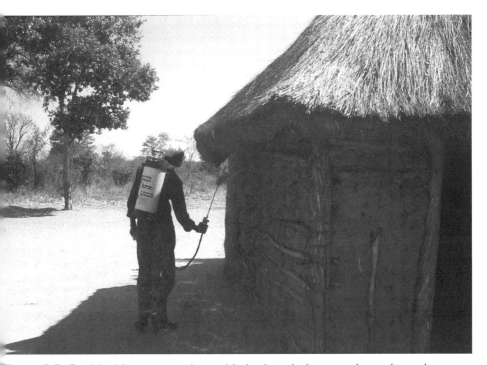

Figure 5.5: Residual house spraying – this is done indoors and, as shown here, under the eaves

covered, while avoiding supporting poles, large pieces of furniture and other obstacles. In Tanzania, it was found that an experienced spray trainer could train men and women from local communities to spray to an acceptable standard in a few days. The villagers needed a refresher course when houses needed respraying six months later. Since access is often a problem when outside teams conduct spraying, employing local villagers made access to all houses much easier.

Community support is needed in IRS programmes and many programmes fail because this is neglected. Most of the communication with communities is done by spray team supervisors and their managers, and community concerns must be considered in operational planning.

Insecticide formulations

Insecticides for house spraying are generally purchased as water-dispersible or wettable powders (WP), or sometimes in micro-encapsulated (CS) or emulsifiable concentrate (EC) formulations. All of these are mixed with an appropriate volume of water to achieve the optimum dosage of active ingredient (a.i.) shown in Table 5.2 (page 152).

For example: to achieve 2 gm DDT/m^2 from a WP that contains 50% active ingredient, requires 2/0.5 = 4 gm WP/ 50 ml (the volume to be sprayed per m^2).

A spray pump with an 8 litre (8000 ml) capacity requires 4 × 8000/50 = 640 gm of WP. The amount can be weighed out once and its volume marked on a suitable container, which is then used as a measure for the powder.

The correct amount of the WP formulation is then thoroughly mixed with the required volume of water in a bucket, and the suspension is poured into the spray pump. Alternatively pre-measured sachets, or the appropriate volume of a liquid concentrate such as CS, can be placed directly into the pump, adding water up to the eight litre mark and swirling the pump contents to mix them.

Comparison of ITNs and IRS

In recent comparative trials, the impact on malaria of insecticide-treated mosquito nets (ITNs) and indoor residual spraying (IRS) has been fairly similar. However, the amount of insecticide needed to treat enough nets for a family is very much less than that required to spray the walls and ceiling of a house. Using less insecticide means that the cost per family protected can be lower (even considering the cost of the net itself), if the nets are delivered in a cost-effective way. In addition, spraying requires equipment and trained people, whereas net treatment campaigns are operationally less demanding.

Mosquitoes are attracted to people sleeping under nets, so applying insecticide to nets may be considered a more targeted approach to killing mosquitoes. In villages where treated nets are widely used, this can result in a reduction of the adult mosquito population. Another advantage of nets is that they can be used over beds, or whatever a person sleeps on, inside or outside the house. In this way, people who sleep outside – such as those who sleep near their crops to guard them, or those who just prefer to sleep outside when it is very hot – can be protected. Nevertheless, comparison of the results of some house spraying projects in Africa in the 1950s, 1960s and 1970s shows that better results were achieved than any so far achieved with ITNs. In addition, treated materials and house spraying both repel and/or kill other household pests such as bedbugs.

In view of the evidence that ITNs are generally effective in a wide range of circumstances, high ITN coverage must always be seen as a desirable programme goal. Whether IRS can be used as an alternative or addition to ITNs needs careful consideration based on country circumstances.

Control of mosquito larvae

Preventive programmes involving insecticidal control of adult mosquitoes are, on the whole, more effective at reducing malaria transmission than those involving larval control. For this reason, the control of mosquito larvae has a lower priority than control of the adult mosquito. It needs more time and specialised knowledge to apply, and is not appropriate in many important environments, particularly in rural areas. However, it may be useful in specific, limited environments, as described below.

Targeting breeding sites

In most places, only one or two of the local *Anopheles* species are important malaria vectors. Although most *Anopheles* malaria vectors breed in natural or man-made bodies of surface water, which are usually located in open countryside, each *Anopheles* species has a characteristic range of preferred breeding sites (see Box 5.2; also Chapter 1, page 16).

Box 5.2 Species and breeding sites

Species	Preferred breeding sites
Anopheles darlingi	slow-moving rivers
Anopheles minimus	foothill streams and ditches
Anopheles umbrosus	complete shade
Anopheles gambiae	typically small, numerous and shifting, such as small rain-puddles and hoof prints
Anopheles albimanus	typically small, numerous and shifting, such as small rain-puddles and hoof prints
Anopheles stephensi	wells and water tanks

Some mosquito species prefer specific locations that are relatively stable and easy to identify; others are less selective and breed in a range of sites. Sites to be targeted, therefore, vary from region to region.

It is more difficult to sustain effective larval control where breeding sites are small, numerous and shifting, such as in rural areas of Africa. Moreover, larval control is made more difficult by the fact that adult female mosquitoes are capable of flying quite long distances (several kilometres) from breeding sites to find sources of blood. This means that breeding must be thoroughly eliminated over large areas in order to produce effective control. In Africa, larval control is only regarded as a cost-effective intervention in *some* urban environments. This is because most potential urban breeding habitats are either enclosed in concrete or polluted – and hence unsuitable for *Anopheles*. Those that are not, usually sites of urban cultivation, are fixed and easy to identify.

There are few situations where vector breeding is not influenced by human activities and many where man-made breeding sites are important. Some people consider the creation of mosquito breeding sites as a form of environmental pollution. Although it may be impossible to remove every breeding site, it is important to increase the awareness of the community and to ensure that human activities do not inadvertently worsen the situation.

Community views and participation

Larval control programmes should seek the assistance of people who are experienced in searching for larvae and identifying them.

Do not assume that the community always has an accurate knowledge of where the important breeding sites for malaria vectors are. Many community-based environmental actions aimed at 'getting rid of mosquitoes and malaria' are poorly targeted for this reason. Health professionals are often not sufficiently well trained in vector biology to guide communities in effective targeting.

Community participation in vector control, when initiated by public health authorities has been difficult to sustain in many situations because large-scale communal action is required over a wide area for success. It is only worthwhile taking action if all or most households participate.

Targeting breeding sites of different genera

If you work in a malaria control programme, it is important that you are fully aware of the distinction between *Anopheles, Culex* and *Aedes* breeding sites. Without this knowledge there is a danger that you will spend disproportionate amounts of resources on the easily found *Culex* and *Aedes* sites, and leave the harder to find but medically more important *Anopheles* unattended. The control of *Culex* and *Aedes* is nonetheless important in many areas, because the adults can transmit filariasis and dengue respectively. The control of the nuisance from the biting of these genera of mosquito may also be an important priority to the public, who

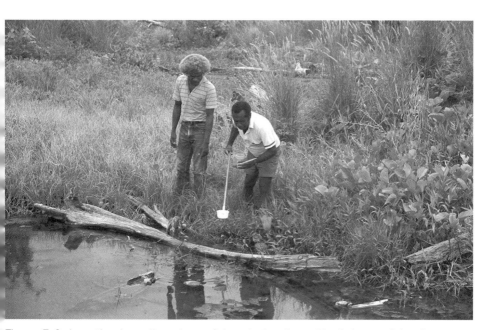

Figure 5.6: Locating breeding sites of *Anopheles farauti* in Solomon Islands

may not make a distinction between mosquito nuisance and the malaria threat.

Culex quinquefasciatus larvae are found in organically polluted water in open drains, cesspits and pit latrines. *Aedes aegypti* larvae are found in water pots, jars and rain-filled garbage. Note also that *Anopheles* larvae float parallel to the water surface whereas *Culex* and *Aedes* hang at an angle from the surface. (For more information on *Anopheles* breeding sites, see Chapter 1, page 16.)

Box 5.3 Steps in targeting breeding sites

> If you are to target malaria vector breeding sites effectively, you need to follow these five steps:
>
> 1 Identify important malaria vectors in the area.
> 2 Find out the breeding habits of these malaria vectors.
> 3 Locate all potential breeding sites (within a radius of up to 2 km, and preferably 4 km, in rural areas).
> 4 Target the most productive breeding sites.
> 5 Divide the target area into sections and assign responsibility for action.

Attacking breeding sites

Attacks on breeding sites must always be thorough. This is because the impact of larval control on malaria transmission is related to the proportion of breeding sites that are dealt with effectively. Your target area must be large enough to include all breeding sites that make a significant contribution to the local adult mosquito population. Attacking breeding sites is usually relatively straightforward once you have found them. Finding all the sites that need to be dealt with is often more difficult.

In any given area, it is not usually necessary to apply larval control to every single body of water. In most places, many bodies of water can be ruled out because they are never sites for malaria vector breeding, and many others can be given low priority since vector breeding in them is rare. Of the sites where vector breeding is relatively common, some will be much more productive than others. Appropriate targeting is, therefore, essential – and, as already mentioned, targeting is a highly species-specific operation. Local surveys, which usually need to be repeated in different seasons, are very useful. Record the findings on a sketch map, if possible, and use them to guide priorities for control.

In larval control operations, a common procedure is to divide the target area into sections. The workforce is then divided into teams, with each team responsible for a section. This enables the team to get to know their specific area and the people living there. Potential breeding sites should be visited at weekly intervals to ensure that new breeding sites are identified quickly and dealt with in time to prevent the emergence of adult mosquitoes.

Methods of attacking breeding sites

Larvae can be killed by using oils, synthetic insecticides, including pyrethroids, insect growth regulators, bacterial insecticide or some natural plant products. Biological and environmental controls are also worth investigating. However, there is no evidence that the removal of bush or cutting grass is effective in controlling mosquitoes.

Larviciding

Oils

Oils have been used as larvicides for many years. They are safe and effective in small enclosed breeding sites, but are messy and only temporarily effective.

Synthetic insecticides

These insecticides are effective, but cannot be used in many breeding sites because most *Anopheles* species breed in water that might be used for bathing, cooking or drinking. Of the conventional insecticides available, the organophosphate **temephos** (Abate®) is the preferred option. It is effective and safe in drinking water, if used at a concentration of one part per million. In most parts of the world *Anopheles* species remain fully susceptible. However, resistance is found in nuisance-biting *Culex quinquefasciatus* and in some populations of the dengue vector *Aedes aegypti*.

Pyrethroids

Pyrethroids are expensive and are very toxic to fish, and so are not suitable for larviciding.

Insect growth regulators

These substances are much safer for vertebrates. However, with some insect growth regulators, mosquito larvae do not die immediately after treatment: they remain alive and motile for some days, but fail to pupate. This makes operational quality control more difficult. However, a study in Sri Lankan gem pits showed that retreatment with insect growth regulator was only needed twice a year, in comparison to temephos or oil which needed reapplying twelve times.

Bacterial insecticide

Bacillus thuringiensis H-14 (BTI), a bacterial insecticide, is even more environmentally benign than insect growth regulators, because it is only toxic to mosquitoes and blackfly *Simulium* larvae. BTI can be very effective, but it is not always the most cost-effective option, and the residual action against surface-feeding *Anopheles* is often very short.

Natural products

In India, products derived from the neem tree, *Azadirachta indica*, which is common in many parts of the tropics, have proved to be very effective for larviciding in rice fields. There have been many laboratory studies on plant products with larvicidal action, but regrettably few have been carried on to extensive field trials.

Applying larvicide

Pressurised spray pumps, like those used for house spraying, can be used to deliver dilute insecticide (see page 156). However, granular formulations of larvicides may be preferable. Although they can be bulkier to transport, these formulations are easier to handle and penetrate better into water covered by emergent vegetation. You can make 'home-made' granular formulations by soaking liquid formulations into small pieces of corncob or coconut husk shortly before application.

Application rates for larvicides are normally specified in terms of the area, rather than the volume, of the water in which you want to prevent breeding. The assumption is usually made that the water is 10 cm deep.

Biological control

Biological control is an attractive approach because it is less risky to humans and is less harmful to the environment than other control methods. In practice, however, it is difficult. There are few examples of effective malaria control using biological methods. Most success stories have involved using vector-eating fish and have been in situations where almost all adult vector mosquitoes breed in a single well-defined category of site – such as rice fields in China, or wells and ponds in villages in Karnataka State, India. The most widely used fish are the top minnow *Gambusia affinis* and the guppy *Poecilia reticulata*.

Environmental control

The range of possible environmental interventions is very wide. It includes permanent and temporary alterations to the environment, ranging from filling and draining breeding sites to planting or removing trees. This makes it difficult to give general recommendations, except when vector species are particularly selective in their breeding habitat preferences and action can be directed at a few well-defined sites.

Filling and draining

Some breeding sites can simply be filled with soil or gravel. On a small scale, this can be done by hand, but larger sites may require the use of mechanical diggers. Sometimes it is easier to drain the site, by constructing open drains or even sub-soil drains. This type of operation requires planning and, where possible, the assistance of an engineer. For more detailed instructions, and suggestions on how to deal with sites ranging from peri-domestic containers to large swamps, refer to the WHO *Manual on larval control operations in malaria programmes* (WHO, 1973) and a more recent book by Rozendaal (WHO, 1997).

Constructing small dams

Other stream-breeding vectors in Southeast Asia have been controlled by the construction of small dams fitted with automatic siphons. These work by blocking the flow until a certain head of water has built up behind the dam, then suddenly releasing it, so that breeding sites downstream are flushed away. If you are planning to implement interventions such as this, that depend on regular repeated action rather than a permanent modification to the environment, they must be performed at intervals of less than a week in order to prevent any larvae from completing their development.

'Opportunistic' interventions

A common feature of many successful environmental control operations is the imaginative use of local resources. For example, surveys in a small logging town on the Pacific coast of Colombia suggested that the breeding of the main local vector, *Anopheles albimanus*, was confined to a few well-defined ponds and pits. Meanwhile in the same town, large quantities of gravel were being dredged from the local river by the logging company to make roads. By diverting a small fraction of this gravel, the ponds were filled, and breeding in them was completely and permanently prevented. Other similar 'opportunistic' interventions have been devised by a series of projects in India.

Control of larvae in rice fields

In some cases, such as rice fields, vector breeding sites are obvious, simple to locate and accessible, but too big to deal with easily. In some areas, including South and Southeast Asia, the anopheline species in the rice fields tend not to be important malaria vectors, although malaria vector species may be found in the streams and channels surrounding the fields. However, in China, Africa and parts of Latin America, malaria vectors breed in the rice fields themselves.

As yet, no universally feasible method has been found to prevent this and more research is needed into methods of rice cultivation that do not result in vector breeding. One method, intermittent irrigation, where fields are drained dry every few days, can be very successful. It does not usually reduce the rice yield, but requires the soil to be sufficiently porous to allow complete drying.

Bioenvironmental control

The aim of 'bioenvironmental control' is to select a pragmatic combination of environmental and biological interventions that:

- are sustainable and adapted to local circumstances
- are integrated with or carried out alongside other local developmental activities
- have other benefits for the community.

Varying degrees of success have been achieved, depending on local circumstances. Examples of these interventions include land-reclamation through filling and draining, and the conversion of breeding sites into fish cultivation ponds. The key elements of this approach involve promoting close collaboration between the community, experts and local authorities; considering local priorities in decision-making, and emphasising sustainability.

The grass-cutting myth

A widespread myth, particularly in Africa, is that cutting down the grass and bush around houses will help to control mosquitoes, especially malaria vectors. In many cases, this is taken to include the destruction of crops such as maize. Since bush-cutting is a relatively easy task, it tends to divert efforts away from mosquito control activities that are actually effective but more difficult. *There is no evidence that grass and maize are breeding sites for any kind of mosquito, or that the removal of bush to deprive mosquitoes of daytime resting sites is effective.*

Key points

> ▶ Malaria can be prevented through the use of insecticidal control of adult *Anopheles* mosquitoes, through protecting humans from mosquito bites, and by reducing mosquito breeding.
>
> ▶ ITN programmes have been implemented since the 1980s but now need to be scaled up to national level.
>
> ▶ Insecticide eventually washes off nets and needs to be re-applied, except in the case of good quality manufactured long-lasting insecticidal nets.
>
> ▶ Indoor residual spraying is effective but logistically demanding.
>
> ▶ Larvae can be killed by using oils, synthetic insecticides, insect growth regulators, bacterial insecticide or some plant products, but larval control is not of such widespread utility as adult mosquito control.
>
> ▶ Biological interventions are possible but there is no evidence that the removal of bush or cutting of grass is effective in controlling mosquitoes.

Further reading

1 Rozendaal, J.A. *Vector control: Methods for use by individuals and communities*, WHO Geneva, 1997
2 Roll Back Malaria, Ed. *Insecticide-treated mosquito net interventions: a manual for national control programme managers*, WHO Geneva, 2003

6 ► Malaria in Pregnancy

Bernard Brabin

This chapter describes:

► what happens when a woman gets malaria during her pregnancy

► the epidemiology of malaria in pregnancy

► the risks associated with HIV and malaria in pregnancy.

It discusses:

► how to manage malaria and anaemia in pregnant women

► ways of preventing malaria in pregnant women

► supportive interventions for controlling malaria.

It will be useful for primary health care workers, and health workers at different levels of health facility.

Introduction

Malaria in pregnancy, particularly *P. falciparum* malaria, is a serious health problem. It is possibly the most important cause of low birth weight in infants of **primigravidae** (i.e. mothers bearing their first child) in highly malarious areas. Low birth weight and stillbirth were recognised as complications of malaria during pregnancy more than 50 years ago. An African study in the 1940s also found that pregnant women were more susceptible to *P. falciparum* infection than non-pregnant women. However, it was not until 1956 that the higher incidence of low birth weight and increased *P. falciparum* parasite prevalence was shown to affect primigravidae more than **multigravidae**.

It is still not completely clear why pregnancy is associated with an increased risk of malaria infection. We do know that pregnancy alters the mother's immune system, making her less likely to reject the fetus – and this may make her more vulnerable to infections such as malaria. The lack of antibodies which prevent *P. falciparum* malaria parasites from adhering to the placenta is also a factor.

Adverse outcomes of malaria in pregnancy

Malaria infection during pregnancy has adverse consequences on the health of the mother, the fetus and the newborn.

The mother

The clinical impact of malaria in pregnancy on maternal health may range from negligible to severe. It will depend, to a great extent, on the immune status of the mother. Acquired anti-malarial immunity depends on the intensity of transmission of malaria, the number of previous pregnancies and the presence of other conditions that decrease immunity such as HIV infection. Adverse outcomes of pregnancy that malaria infection can either directly cause, or significantly contribute to, include: parasitaemia, splenomegaly, anaemia, fever, cerebral malaria, hypoglycaemia, **puerperal** sepsis, pulmonary oedema, haemorrhage and death.

Some women recover more slowly from malaria infection during pregnancy. This may lead to a longer duration and raised prevalence of parasitaemia (the presence of parasites in the blood). This, in turn, may be associated with an increased incidence of clinical malaria, although many pregnant women living in areas of high transmission remain asymptomatic (i.e. they have parasites in their blood, but do not show any significant symptoms of malaria).

A reduction in parasite prevalence usually occurs late in pregnancy. This is not related to the use of anti-malarial drugs. It partly relates to parasites being 'sequestered' ('hiding') in the placenta rather than in the blood, so that they do not show up on blood slides. It also results from the mother developing immunity to the malaria parasite during her pregnancy.

Pregnant women are more likely to be anaemic than non-pregnant women. Even those with apparently asymptomatic infections may be anaemic. Malaria contributes substantially to anaemia in pregnant women, as do other factors such as HIV infection, inadequate nutrition, **haemoglobinopathies**, and **hookworm** infection. The incidence and prevalence of maternal anaemia (haemoglobin less than eleven grams per decilitre, or < 11 gmdl^{-1}) and severe anaemia (haemoglobin less than seven grams per decilitre, or < 7 gmdl^{-1}) is higher in first pregnancies than in later pregnancies in women living in malarious areas. This is a consequence of the increased malaria parasite prevalence and the severity of infection in primigravidae.

In highly endemic areas, it is unclear how much low birth weight and pre-term delivery are due to malaria-related anaemia and how much to parasitaemia. This is because parasitaemia is always accompanied by some degree of malarial anaemia. In addition, anaemia caused by inadequate nutrition tends to be highly prevalent in malarious areas. However, studies from Papua New Guinea suggest that malaria plays a greater role in causing low birth weight than nutritional anaemia. The risk of women dying from malaria in pregnancy increases with the development of severe anaemia. Mortality is especially high during epidemics.

The fetus

If a woman is infected with malaria during her pregnancy, this can result in abortion, stillbirth, congenital infection or anaemia in the unborn child. The risk of these outcomes is higher in areas of low or epidemic malaria transmission (see page 171). Maternal anaemia and malaria infection during the second trimester both reduce weight gain in the fetus.

The infant

Malaria can cause the fetus to grow more slowly (intrauterine growth restriction, IUGR) and thus result in a low birth weight (less than 2500 gms). The cells of placentas infected with *P. falciparum* parasites change in characteristic ways that we think inhibit fetal growth. An infected placenta is less efficient at transferring maternal antibodies to the fetus, and this can weaken the infant's immunity. In areas of high malaria transmission, up to 60% of low birth weight in first pregnancies may be due to malaria. Low birth weight is an important risk factor for neonatal and early infant mortality. Mortality in low birth weight infants is much higher than mortality in normal birth weight infants.

Malaria epidemiology and malaria in pregnancy

The clinical features of *P. falciparum* malaria in pregnancy depend upon transmission levels.

High to moderate transmission areas

People living in both highly and moderately endemic areas develop partial immunity to malaria. This immunity is altered during pregnancy. Infection is frequently asymptomatic and therefore may not be suspected. A woman's immunity during pregnancy depends on the number of children she has had (is 'parity specific'). The fewer the children (or the lower the parity), the lower the level of immunity to malaria during the pregnancy. There may also be an absence of parasites in the bloodstream, because they have become sequestered in the placenta. This means that even if her blood test is microscope negative, you should not exclude the possibility of malaria in a pregnant woman.

Malaria in pregnancy in high and moderate transmission areas can also cause anaemia, which may be severe in the mother and result in low birth weight in the baby. The risk of anaemia in both mother and baby is higher in first and second pregnancies than in later pregnancies. Severe anaemia may develop slowly over several weeks, and may be associated with iron and folate deficiency. Many women can tolerate relatively severe anaemia if it is of slow onset, compared to rapid onset when tolerance is poor.

Low transmission and epidemic prone areas

In areas of low transmission or during epidemics, the population will not have significant levels of malaria immunity. There will therefore be no parity-specific differences in immunity. In such areas, malaria infection in pregnancy means a very high risk of both maternal and **perinatal** mortality. Non-immune pregnant women are likely to be more severely ill than women who are not pregnant, and their condition will deteriorate more rapidly. These women need to be treated speedily, using a protocol which is known to be effective. Symptoms on presentation may include hyperpyrexia, hypoglycaemia, severe haemolytic anaemia, cerebral malaria and pulmonary oedema.

In Africa, some cities have lower malaria transmission than rural areas. This places young urban women at greater risk of pregnancy complications and maternal death. Malaria-related maternal morbidity in adolescents in towns and cities is therefore likely to be underestimated.

A summary of the complications of malaria in pregnancy for both the mother and the fetus in high and low transmission areas is shown in Table 6.1.

Table 6.1: Maternal and fetal effects of malaria in pregnancy

Maternal or fetal effect	First pregnancies in areas with stable malaria	All pregnancies in areas with unstable malaria
High maternal fever	+	+++
Severe maternal malaria		
Severe anaemia	+++	+++
Cerebral malaria	–	++
Hypoglycaemia	+	++
Pulmonary oedema	–	++
Acute renal failure	–	++
Placental infection	+++	++
Puerperal sepsis	++	++
Low birth weight	+++	+++
IUGR	++	+
Prematurity	+	++
Abortion and stillbirth	+	++
Congenital malaria	+	+
Fetal anaemia (cord Hb < 12.5 g/dl)	+	+

+++   very common
++   common
+   infrequent
–   rare
IUGR intrauterine growth restriction

Other malaria species

Studies in Thailand and India reported that *P. vivax* malaria during pregnancy is associated with maternal anaemia and low birth weight, but to a lesser degree than *P. falciparum*.

HIV and malaria in pregnancy

Human immunodeficiency virus (HIV) infection reduces a pregnant woman's ability to control *P. falciparum* infection. HIV is therefore associated with a significant increase in malaria prevalence in pregnant women of all parities. If a woman is infected with HIV, parity will not affect the risks associated with placental infection because HIV infection appears to restrict the development of parity-specific immunity. We do not yet fully understand the immunological mechanisms involved.

Women with HIV infection are more likely to have symptomatic infections and to have an increased risk of malaria with adverse birth outcomes. Higher prevalence of malaria in HIV-infected pregnant women of all parities increases the risk of low birth weight. In pregnant women HIV also independently increases the risk of both maternal anaemia and low birth weight. The effect of HIV on malaria prevalence is apparent from before 20 weeks gestation. This has been observed in studies in Malawi and in western Kenya.

Control of malaria in pregnancy

The control of malaria in pregnancy requires a multi-intervention approach, including effective case management of malaria, the use of **intermittent preventive treatment (IPT)** (depending upon endemicity of malaria – see page 179), and the use of insecticide-treated mosquito nets (ITNs). The proportion of women using IPT or ITNs are useful indicators for monitoring malaria control in pregnancy. For best results from these interventions, a good education strategy is essential, so that pregnant women are fully aware of the increased risks of malaria and the best ways to reduce the risk.

In many places, a malaria control programme for pregnant women may already exist, but its effectiveness may be unknown. In order to assess the extent of the problem of malaria in pregnancy *and* to measure the impact of interventions, it is important to identify appropriate indicators (for example, low birth weight babies, maternal anaemia, etc.).

Assessing the extent of the problem

Low birth weight is *potentially* the most useful indicator of the extent of the problem because the effect of malaria in pregnancy on birth weight is so sensitive and specific. It has, therefore, been proposed that the number of low birth weight babies in primigravidae compared to multigravidae can be used as an indicator of the effectiveness of measures to control malaria in pregnancy. Because of the importance of low birth weight for child survival, another useful indicator could be neonatal mortality, although this is more difficult to determine and interpret. As discussed above, in areas of low transmission, the case fatality rate would be an important indicator. In addition, new methods using maternal anaemia as a malaria control indicator are being developed.

In order to compare the ratio of low birth weight infants in primigravidae and in multigravidae, the first step is to gather the data needed for this comparison. This is usually only available from health centre and hospital delivery books. A useful form of tally sheet for recording from delivery books is shown in Figure 6.1.

Box 6.1: Tally method for recording low birth weights

- Check that both birth weight values and the mother's parity are recorded in the delivery book.
- Record the number of low birth weight (< 2500 gm) and normal birth weight babies (≥ 2500 gm) for first pregnancies and for later pregnancies (see example tally sheet, Table 6.2).
- These may be recorded using two separate tally sheets, one for primigravidae and the other for multigravidae.
- The year of delivery should be noted and the tallies recorded by month, if possible.

Figure 6.1: Examples of tally sheets

Sheet One: Primigravidae (first pregnancies)   Year:

Low birth weight (< 2500 gm)	Normal birth weight (≥ 2500 gm)
January ~~1111~~ ~~1111~~ ~~1111~~ etc	~~1111~~ ~~1111~~ ~~1111~~ ~~1111~~ etc.
February	
March	
↓	↓

Sheet Two: Multigravidae (all later pregnancies 2, 3, 4, 5 → etc.)   Year:

Low birth weight (< 2500 gm)	Normal birth weight (≥ 2500 gm)
January ~~1111~~ ~~1111~~ ~~1111~~ etc	~~1111~~ ~~1111~~ ~~1111~~ ~~1111~~ etc.
February	
March	
↓	↓

When the tallies have been counted, you can calculate the odds ratio (OR) of low birth weight risk in primigravidae compared with multigravidae. When you are using such data, calculations of OR should be made over at least the preceding two years, using a sample size of at least 500 (about 100 primigravidae and 400 multi-gravidae). The method for calculating this ratio is shown using an example in Table 6.2.

Table 6.2: Tally sheet for recording from delivery books

	Primigravidae	Multigravidae
Number of low birth weights recorded	30 = A	40 = C
Number of normal birth weights recorded	70 = B	360 = D
	100	400
Odds Ratio = $\frac{A \times D}{B \times C} = \frac{30 \times 360}{70 \times 40} = 3.86$		

Values over 1.7 are likely to indicate a significant amount of malaria in pregnancy. Values over 2.5 would indicate a high level of malaria exposure with poor malaria control. Values less than 1.5 would suggest good levels of malaria control in pregnancy have been achieved. Note, however, that values based on data from health facilities may not be representative of the entire community, because not all women deliver in health centres or hospitals. This method should be applied in assessments in Africa.

Effective case management of malaria in pregnancy

Anti-malarials drugs may be used for treatment or prevention. The national policy on first and second-line anti-malarials for the treatment of malaria in pregnancy will depend on levels of parasite resistance to the available drugs. (Drug resistance is discussed further in Chapter 4: The Treatment of Malaria.) It will also depend on the efficacy and safety of the drug for use in pregnancy. *P. falciparum* may not respond as well to anti-malarial treatment in pregnant women as it does in non-pregnant women. Parasites sequestered in the placenta may not be cleared, and this may partly explain why recrudescence is more common in pregnant women.

Any pregnant woman with symptoms of malaria requires immediate treatment. She is at risk of fetal loss, premature delivery or death. The aim of effective management of malaria in pregnant women is not only to cure the clinical symptoms but also to clear all parasites, because even low level parasitaemia presents a risk to both the mother and the fetus. *P. falciparum* parasites may be sequestered in the placenta and not detectable in the peripheral blood. This means that, in malaria endemic areas, you should treat all pregnant women who present with either fever or anaemia with an effective anti-malarial. This includes those with a negative blood slide.

There is no consensus on the optimal anti-malarial regimen for use in pregnancy. The regimen varies from country to country, depending on factors such as levels of resistance, affordability and ease of use. The management of malaria in pregnancy should be part of the national anti-malarial guidelines (see Chapter 4). Where the guidelines are in place, you should always follow them. These guidelines should make clear the safety issues for use of anti-malarials in pregnant women. Some anti-malarials are safe in the second and third trimesters, but not in the first. Always treat uncomplicated symptomatic malaria in the first trimester.

Box 6.2: Anti-malarials to be used in pregnancy

The anti-malarials that are currently recommended for use in pregnancy include:

▶ chloroquine in areas where parasites are still sensitive (primarily for *P. vivax* infection)

▶ sulfadoxine-pyrimethamine (S-P) in areas with parasite resistance to chloroquine and sensitivity to S-P

▶ quinine may be used in areas where parasites are resistant to both chloroquine and S-P.

WHO currently recommends that the following drugs should *not* be used in pregnancy:

▶ halofantrine, tetracycline, doxycycline, and primaquine.

Notes on other anti-malarials

▶ Mefloquine has successfully been used for treatment, but was associated with a slightly increased risk of stillbirths in a study in Thailand.

▶ The artemisinin derivatives have proved useful in areas with multi-drug *resistant P. falciparum* malaria: data on their reproductive toxicity is still being collected.

▶ Artesunate and artemether can be used in second and third trimesters, although data on their toxicity is still required.

▶ There is little published information on amodiaquine in pregnancy, but it can be used in second and third trimesters, if there is no alternative.

Ministry of Health

FLOWCHART ON MALARIA-IN-PREGNANCY

Is the woman pregnant?

YES

If YES, does she have signs and symptoms of malaria?

YES   NO

Treat as SIMPLE MALARIA if she presents with:
- a fever
- shivering, chills, rigors
- sweating
- headaches
- dizziness
- muscle or joint pain
- loss of appetite
- nausea and vomiting
- blood slide of + or ++ MPs

DAY 1:
Give **3 tabs of SP** (Fansidar) + **4 tabs of CQ** (Chloroquine)

DAY 2:
Give **4 tabs of CQ** (Chloroquine)

DAY 3:
Give **2 tabs of CQ** (Chloroquine)
- Review on 3rd day

**OR
REFER**

- *if she is allergic to sulpha drugs, OR*
- *she is below 4 or above 8 months of pregnancy, OR*
- *she doesn't respond to treatment, OR*
- *when you are not sure*

Treat as SEVERE MALARIA if she presents with other signs such as:
- confusion
- convulsions, fits
- drowsiness or coma
- unable to walk unsupported
- anaemia
- jaundice
- temperature $\geq$ 40°C
- vomiting everything
- black urine (coffee-like)
- threatened abortion (uterine contractions and P.V. bleeding)
- blood slide of +++ or ++++ MPs

Give one dose of **i.m. Injection Quinine 10mg/kg BWT.**
(anterior thigh) after diluting with water or saline in ratio of 1:2, then *REFER IMMEDIATELY*

Give 2 doses of **IPT*** as directly observed treatment, i.e.
- **3 tabs of SP** (Fansidar) between the **4th and 6th months** of pregnancy
- **3 tabs of SP** (Fansidar) between the **7th and 8th months** of pregnancy

- *add single doses of **Mebendazole (500mg)** in the same periods/months,*
- ***Iron (FeSo$_4$) 200mg daily,***
- ***Folic acid 5mg daily** (after 1 week of SP administration),*
- *Counsel on **insecticide treated mosquito net (ITN) use and nutrition***

KEY:

IPT = Intermittent Presumptive Treatment

SP = Sulfadoxine-Pyrimethamine

* HIV positive pregnant women should be given at least 3 doses of SP one month apart between 16-36 weeks of pregnancy.

Figure 6.2: Example of flowchart used in Uganda for management of malaria in pregnancy

Management of anaemia in pregnancy

Anaemia poses a great risk both to the pregnant woman and to the fetus, even when the anaemia is not symptomatic. Ideally, you should screen all pregnant women for anaemia at antenatal visits. In malaria endemic areas, treat all anaemic pregnant women with an effective anti-malarial, irrespective of the results of blood microscopy, and irrespective of the presence or absence of fever.

Antenatal iron (ferrous sulphate) and folate (folic acid) supplements should be provided, using nationally recommended doses. There is currently no evidence that iron supplementation in pregnancy can increase malaria recrudescence or that folate supplementation is harmful.

Severe malaria in pregnancy

Severe malaria may occur more in women with little or no immunity, including those who live in areas with low or irregular malaria transmission. Inadequate treatment (for example, because of underdosing or high levels of drug resistance) can contribute to the risk of developing severe malaria. It is more common during malaria epidemics, when mortality is high. Pregnant women are particularly at risk of developing pulmonary oedema and hypoglycaemia. Cerebral malaria is especially common in pregnant adolescents in urban areas. Clinical diagnosis and treatment is similar to that for adults with severe malaria, which you will find described in other chapters in this book.

Prevention of malaria in pregnancy

The prevention of malaria during pregnancy requires chemoprophylaxis or the use of intermittent preventive treatment (IPT), plus the use of insecticide-treated mosquito nets (ITNs). However, it is often not possible to deliver effective chloroquine chemoprophylaxis, because people do not adhere to the treatment regimen. For this reason many countries have adopted IPT. However, WHO–AFRO no longer recommends chemoprophylaxis with chloroquine in pregnant women, because of high levels of drug resistance and frequently poor **compliance**.

Initial treatment dose

In malaria endemic areas, WHO recommends a treatment dose of an anti-malarial for all pregnant women at their first attendance at antenatal clinic. The first treatment dose is given without screening for malaria parasitaemia, and regardless of whether the woman is symptomatic.

Intermittent preventive treatment

WHO recommends that in areas of stable malaria transmission, IPT with an effective anti-malarial drug, preferably one dose, be provided as part of antenatal care. You will need to provide this treatment from the second trimester onwards.

IPT involves the administration of full, curative treatment doses of an effective anti-malarial drug at pre-defined intervals during pregnancy. These are given irrespective of peripheral blood status (that is, whether parasitaemic or not). The treatment doses are given at least one month apart in the second and third trimesters. Currently the drug used for IPT is S-P, because it is safe and easy to administer. It is a one dose (three tablets per dose) treatment, which the pregnant woman can take under your direct observation at the health facility.

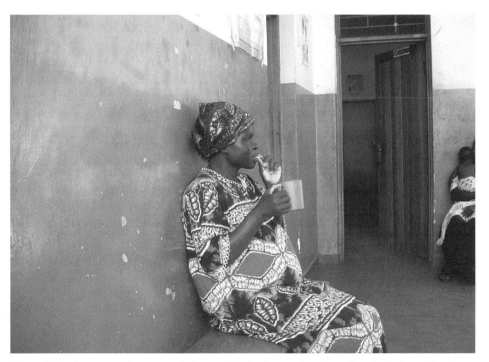

Figure 6.3: A pregnant women takes sulfadoxine-pyrimethamine for intermittent preventive treatment (IPT)

Provision of S-P two or three times in pregnancy at greater than monthly intervals has been shown to be effective in reducing placental parasitaemia, improving birth weight and preventing severe maternal anaemia in primigravidae. Data suggest that women co-infected with HIV require an increased number of monthly doses of S-P during pregnancy. There is evidence of the effectiveness of three doses compared to two. Monthly administration of S-P during the second and third trimesters of pregnancy has been advocated for areas with high HIV prevalence. This should be a policy decision based upon levels of malaria and HIV in the area. Until recently the use of S-P was not recommended after 34 weeks gestation, although there is no good evidence that it is harmful to the fetus after 34 weeks, and if required it can be given after this time.

Insecticide-treated mosquito nets (ITNs)

It is recommended that ITNs are provided to pregnant women as early in pregnancy as possible, and also to adolescent girls before pregnancy. Their use should be encouraged throughout pregnancy and during the postpartum period. ITN use during pregnancy in areas of stable transmission will also provide significant protection against maternal anaemia and low birth weight. The ITN will also protect young infants who sleep with their mother.

Although ITNs may be delivered through any public or private sector distribution method, distribution mechanisms that also help to facilitate the distribution of IPT (in areas of stable malaria transmission), such as through antenatal clinics should be encouraged.

Protection of non-immune pregnant women

We do not have, as yet, any fully effective approaches to ensuring the protection of pregnant women living in areas of low transmission, highly seasonal or epidemic malaria. The use of ITNs, however, should be encouraged. There is no evidence to support the use of IPT. Non-immune pregnant women exposed to malaria require prompt access to treatment of febrile illness. Chemoprophylaxis may be used for prevention in visitors.

Table 6.3: Intervention strategies for malaria during pregnancy, by transmission intensity

	Case management	Intermittent preventive treatment (IPT)	Insecticide-treated nets (ITNs)
High/medium transmission – perennial (stable)*	Risk of febrile illness and severe malaria limited Screen and treat anaemia with recommended anti-malarial drug and iron supplement Promptly recognise and treat all potential malaria illness with an effective drug	Provide pregnant women a standard IPT[1] dose at first regularly scheduled antenatal clinic visit after quickening. At the next routine visit[2], provide an IPT dose, with a minimum of two doses given at not less than a one-month interval[3]	Begin use in adolescents or early in pregnancy and continue postpartum Emphasise including young children sleeping under ITNs
High/medium transmission – seasonal (stable)*	Risk of febrile illness and severe malaria limited Screen and treat anaemia with recommended anti-malarial drug and iron supplement Promptly recognise and treat all potential malaria illness with an effective drug	Provide pregnant women a standard IPT[1] dose at first regularly scheduled antenatal clinic visit after quickening. At the next routine visit[2] provide an IPT dose, with a minimum of two doses given at not less than a one-month interval[3]	Begin use in adolescents or early in pregnancy and continue postpartum Emphasise including young children sleeping under ITNs
Low transmission (unstable)**	Risk of febrile illness, anaemia and severe malaria high Promptly recognise and treat all potential malaria illness with an effective drug Screen and treat anaemia with recommended anti-malarial drug and iron supplement Consider P. vivax infection in East Africa[4]	IPT cannot be recommended in these areas, based on present evidence	Begin use early in pregnancy and continue postpartum Emphasise including young children sleeping under ITNs

[Notes for Table 6.3, page 182]

NOTES:
* Adult women have a high level of acquired anti-malarial immunity; first and second pregnancies are at higher risk of adverse consequences of malaria.
** Adult women have no or very low level of acquired anti-malarial immunity; all pregnancies are at risk of adverse consequences of malaria.
1 Presently the most effective drug for IPT is sulfadoxine-pyrimethamine.
2 WHO recommends an ideal schedule of three antenatal clinic visits after quickening.
3 In areas where HIV prevalence among pregnant women is > 10%, a third dose should be administered at the last scheduled visit. If the pregnant woman had received only one dose at the time of the third visit, a second dose should be administered at the fourth visit.
4 CQ chemoprophylaxis to decrease the burden of *P. vivax* in pregnancy may be considered, but no evidence on effectiveness of this strategy is presently available.

(Source: WHO *A Strategic Framework for Malaria Prevention and Control During Pregnancy in the African Region*. Brazzaville: WHO Regional Office for Africa, 2004. AFR/MAL/04/01 www.afro.who.int/malaria/publications/malaria_in_pregnancy_092004.pdf)

Supportive interventions for effective control

Antenatal care

As discussed above, primigravidae in malaria-endemic areas, particularly adolescents, are at greater risk of pregnancy complications from malaria. You will need to provide good quality antenatal care to ensure positive pregnancy outcomes. In malarious areas, regular antenatal care is associated with improved anti-malarial use and haematinic supplementation, reduced low birth weight and improved haemoglobin levels.

Raising awareness

In highly endemic areas of Africa, where a high proportion of primigravidae are adolescents, the potential to reduce low birth weight through effective malaria control in pregnancy is enormous. However, the main barriers to malaria control in pregnancy are often the lack of availability of effective and feasible anti-malarial drug regimens, and non-attendance at existing clinics. There are millions of women who have little knowledge about the extent of the problem, about available services or about ways of helping themselves.

We need to raise awareness at every level to ensure that national programmes implement effective malaria control in pregnancy using existing cost-effective interventions. Communities need to recognise that malaria in pregnancy is a significant health problem that can be both prevented *and* treated.

Key points

> ▶ Pregnancy increases the risk of malaria infection.
>
> ▶ Malaria infection during pregnancy can cause adverse outcomes for the health of the mother, the fetus and the newborn.
>
> ▶ Malaria contributes significantly to anaemia in pregnant women.
>
> ▶ Malaria can cause the fetus to grow more slowly and be born too soon.
>
> ▶ The risks of malaria in pregnancy vary according to the transmission levels in the area where the pregnant woman lives.
>
> ▶ HIV infection increases malaria prevalence in pregnant women.
>
> ▶ Treat any pregnant woman with the symptoms of malaria immediately.
>
> ▶ In malaria endemic areas, treat any pregnant woman who has anaemia with anti-malarials, regardless of the blood microscopy result.
>
> ▶ IPT during pregnancy and ITN use can help reduce malaria in pregnant women and improve pregnancy outcome.
>
> ▶ Surveillance of low birthweight frequency is a useful way of monitoring malaria control in pregnancy.

Further reading

1 Shulman, C.E., Dorman, E.K., Cutts, F., Kawuondo, K., Bulmer, J.N., Peshu, N., Marsh, K. 'Intermittent sulphadoxine-pyrimethamine to prevent severe anaemia secondary to malaria in pregnancy: a randomised placebo-controlled trial' *Lancet*, 1999, 353: pp 632–636

2 Verhoeff, F.H., Brabin, B.J., Hart, C.A., Chimsuku, L., Kazembe, P., Broadhead, R.L. 'Increased prevalence of malaria in HIV-infected pregnant women and its implications for malaria control' *Tropical Medicine and International Health*, 1999, 4: pp 5–12

3 Ter ter Kuile, F.O., Terlouw, D.J., Phillips-Howard, P.A., Hawley, W.A., Friedman, J.F., Kariuki, S.K., Shi, Y.P., Kolczak, M.S., Lal, A.A., Vulule, J.M., Nahlen, B.L. 'Reduction of malaria during pregnancy by permethrin-treated bed nets in an area of intense perennial malaria transmission in western Kenya' *American Journal of Tropical Medicine and Hygiene*, 2003, 68: pp 50–60

4 Brabin, B.J., Agbaje, S.O.F., Ahmed, Y., Briggs, N.D. 'A birthweight nomogram for Africa as a malaria control indicator' *Annals of Tropical Medicine and Parasitology*, 1999, 93: 547–557

7 Planning and Management

Jane Edmondson

This chapter describes:
▶ the basic elements of planning and implementing malaria control at district level.
It discusses:
▶ the role of planning and management in malaria control.
It will be useful for leaders and members of District Health Teams. It should also be helpful to anyone who plans and manages malaria control and related activities at *any* level, particularly district hospitals, regional or provincial levels immediately above district level, and sub-district levels immediately below.

Introduction

Good management can make a huge difference to the success of health services, malaria control included. Technical knowledge and skills are vital, but teams also need management skills to bring together all the necessary parts – people, knowledge, training, money, materials, facilities and time – and organise them into an active project or programme. Management skills still too rarely feature in training programmes or when new staff are being recruited. Staff at all levels will benefit from having some management skills. Even if they do not manage other people, they need to manage their own time and the resources that they work with. At district level, management will be a very large part of people's work.

Management can mean many things. Box 7.1 below offers a general definition.

Box 7.1: Working definition of management

Management is about identifying and achieving organisational objectives through the deployment of appropriate resources. It involves identifying what needs to be done, as well as organising and supporting others to do the necessary tasks.

The basic elements are the same for any field of work, including malaria control:

▶ Managing people: forming and maintaining teams and partnerships, motivating, developing, appraising performance, consulting, etc.
▶ Managing finances and physical resources: monitoring and controlling the use of resources
▶ Managing operations: maintaining and improving the service provided, **logistics**, etc.
▶ Managing information: ensuring effective gathering, holding, using and exchanging of information
▶ Drawing all these together to solve problems, and to make and implement decisions

Planning

Good planning is the basis of good management. A good plan will be based on:

• involving the right people in the planning process
• developing a shared vision of where you want to be in the longer term
• gathering relevant information
• appraising information in order to define clear and achievable objectives (see Box 7.2, page 190)
• applying a realistic assessment of available resources.

The planning process looks at where you are in terms of a particular issue or issues (in this case, malaria), where you would like to be, and how to get from one to the other.

It is rare that a district will be planning something from nothing. There are likely to be at least some resources and activities for malaria control already in place. The plan may therefore need to cover not just new interventions, but also how you are going to continue and improve – or in some cases stop – existing activities.

It is also rare to plan for malaria separately from everything else. It is more likely that districts will be planning a package of integrated services, of which malaria control will be just one part. The elements of the planning process are, however, the same. Many countries will have district planning guidelines and we do not aim to duplicate these. Instead, the following planning steps cover the particular challenges that malaria presents.

Identify who should be involved in planning

Involving key **stakeholders** from the beginning will help foster a shared vision that can be sustained through the planning and **implementation** of malaria control activities. There are some techniques, such as **stakeholder analysis**, for identifying important groups to involve. Questions to ask in deciding who should be involved in planning could include:

- Who is in touch with the practical problems of malaria in households, communities and lower level health facilities?
- Who makes decisions about policies, regulations or resource allocations that may affect implementation of malaria control interventions?
- Who has skills in planning, budgeting, particular interventions, etc.?
- Who has resources that could be used for implementation?
- Who has an overview, for example of district services generally or of malaria nationally?

People can be involved in many ways: as members of a planning team (which may cover more than malaria); on a committee that oversees the team's work; through surveys, interviews, **focus groups, participatory rural appraisal,** or requests for written comments and advice.

Depending on the local situation, possible groups to involve include:

- key decision makers and managers in the district
- community members (particularly representing vulnerable groups)
- whoever will lead implementation
- health workers at different levels of facilities and different cadres (for example **community health workers,** nurses, laboratory staff, doctors)
- representatives of NGOs, faith-based organisations, private sector organisations, research groups and other current or potential partners in malaria in the district
- technical experts at district level, or from elsewhere if the necessary technical expertise is not available in the district
- planning experts at district level

- Ministry of Health officials – planning experts or technical experts
- representatives of potential funding sources.

The planning and implementation cycle

The following sections discuss the management process by examining the different stages of a planning and implementation cycle (as shown in Figure 7.1). This is often referred to simply as a planning cycle, but covers implementation, **monitoring** and **evaluation** as well. Note that the different stages shown in Figure 7.1 are not discrete steps: in practice they will often overlap and feed into each other.

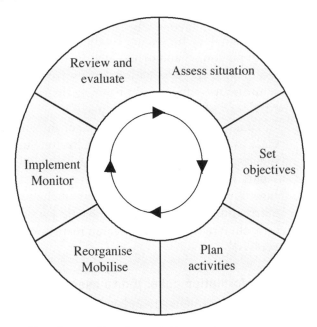

Figure 7.1: Planning and implementation cycle

Assess the situation

Collect information

An early step is to gather information to help assess the malaria situation. You need to decide what this information should be, and how much information is needed.

There needs to be a balance between gathering good quality information and advice, and getting on with implementation. Those involved in planning will certainly need some data on the current situation, both to inform the planning and to support a case for funding. Other chapters in this book can provide ideas on the different kinds of information you could collect: epidemiology, environmental factors, **demography**, socio-economic factors, current health services, current and potential resources (financial, human and physical).

Some of the information needed will already be available. Often, however, it will not be; or, if it is available, it may be of poor quality. You need to decide how much time and money should be spent on collecting information. Many things cannot be measured exactly, or at least not without considerable investment in time and money (for example the precise incidence of malaria in the community). Use data that are already available, or quick and easy to obtain, bearing in mind that there are bound to be some gaps and uncertainties. Districts can plan, appraise and make decisions using such data, backed up by the expertise and experience of local health personnel and others involved in malaria control. You may also be able to get a national view from the Ministry of Health or information from neighbouring districts, and use this together with local information and expertise.

Plans can also be made to collect information that is not currently available, but will be in the future. Such information should be relevant to objectives and relatively simple to obtain (ideally as part of normal working practice) and the cost should be in reasonable proportion to the cost of the whole plan. Where key information is missing, there may be a need for some operational research. Are there local research institutions which could become involved?

Use information collected to assess needs

Information collected can be used to assess needs, to take a critical look at current activities, and to assess potential malaria control activities for the future. Terms and techniques used to assess the situation vary, and include **situation analysis**, start-up analysis, **rapid appraisal** or **needs assessment**. Possible questions should focus on what is needed and what is currently being done.

What is needed?

- What are the major risk factors for malaria in the district?
- Where is the burden greatest: what areas and population groups are at highest risk?
- What specific interventions are appropriate for each area or group? Which of these interventions are likely to have most impact?

What is currently being done?

- How are malaria control activities currently planned and managed?
- Are there clear objectives and a clear vision?
- Who is involved in planning and implementation?
- What is the cost? Is the share of resources that has been allocated to malaria appropriate?
- Is priority given to those areas and population groups at highest risk?
- Do staff have adequate skills, resources and equipment?
- What has been the impact of current activities on malaria deaths and illness? If current activities are not having the desired effect, why is this? What, realistically, can be done about existing problems?
- What research, monitoring and evaluation are currently under way? Do these answer the questions that have been asked?

Set objectives, outputs and activities

Having assessed the situation, it should be possible to identify (a) what is not being done that should be done, and (b) what current activities could be done better, are not useful or not needed. At this stage, it is important to develop a shared vision of how stakeholders would like things to be in the long term. There is likely to be a big difference between what ideally could be done with unlimited resources, and what can be done now with the resources available. It may be possible to do more in the future by raising additional funds, by finding new partners and by building **capacity** in the community, but this will usually take time. Meanwhile, there may be things that can be done differently with the resources already available. For example, resources could be shifted from one method for promoting messages about ITNs to another method that reaches more people more effectively for the same cost. Such considerations will help identify achievable short-term, medium-term and long-term objectives that lead towards the overall purpose, and make it important to include fund-raising and partnership-building activities in short-term plans.

A description of planning terms is given in Box 7.2.

Box 7.2: Planning terms

Different organisations tend to use slightly different terms for planning. But the following are fairly widespread:

Goal
the wider objective(s) which the programme of work will help achieve – the longer term impact (for example to improve the health and well-being of the population in the district)

Purpose
the intended effect(s) for which the programme is directly responsible (for example to reduce the malaria burden in the District) – the essential motivation for the programme

Objectives
what the programme of work needs to achieve in particular areas of work in order to fulfil its purpose, (for example objectives on case management, ITN coverage, behaviour change)

Outputs
what outputs (deliverables) need to be produced in order to achieve a particular objective (for example, all nurses to be trained to treat malaria)

Targets
These are more precise restatements of the goal, purpose or objectives that show, in a measurable way, what the programme aims to have achieved by a fixed point in time (these can be broken down further into very specific measures to be used as **indicators** of progress)

Milestones
These are interim markers of progress on the way to achieving an output or objective and its associated target – a statement of something that should have been done by a fixed point in time

Priorities and objectives

Setting objectives and outputs, particularly in the short term, means being clear about priorities. For malaria this involves appraising the possible malaria control interventions and delivery mechanisms, and selecting the most urgent and important. Criteria for selection will depend on the context, but may include efficacy, resources required, feasibility, acceptability – in other words, factors that will affect the likelihood of achieving impact. Districts may also need to decide which population groups or geographical areas should be given priority. Criteria here may include burden of disease, levels of poverty and current access to services. You may not be able to tackle all the high priorities straightaway. An illustration of this is given in Box 7.3.

Box 7.3: Appraising options: an illustration

A district has identified two major needs: to train health workers in case management and to introduce a promotion scheme for ITNs. The district does not have enough resources to do both now, or at least not throughout the district. They could decide to do both, but only in some parts of the district, or they could decide to do just one throughout the district, and do the rest in later years. The district needs to assess which option or combination of options is likely to have the bigger impact in terms of effectiveness, cost, feasibility, etc. Decisions will depend on the information available (for example, on existing levels of training, existing knowledge about and use of ITNs, levels of morbidity and mortality in different parts of the district) and on judgements about the likely benefits of each option.

In practice, the decisions will probably be more complicated than this example. The important thing is to use the information and opinions collected and then be decisive.

This chapter does not go into detail on setting objectives, outputs, targets, indicators, etc., as this is generally well covered in district guidelines and other texts. However, an example dealing with severe malaria is given in Box 7.4. Clearly the specific objectives in any one district will depend on local circumstances. This shows how several short-term objectives contribute to one or more medium-term objectives which, in turn, contribute to an overall purpose. It also gives examples of related targets (more information on defining targets and indicators is given in the section on monitoring and evaluation).

Clearly these objectives could be broken down into detailed outputs and activities with associated targets and indicators, and could be set alongside objectives on other aspects of malaria control (for example, ITNs, behaviour change) under an overall purpose (for example, to reduce the malaria burden).

Box 7.4: Examples of objective-setting: severe malaria

Objective	Targets
Ten-year objective: – to reduce malaria case fatality rates in **district hospitals**	– malaria case fatality rates reduced by x% compared with current levels by year aaaa
Five-year objectives: – to ensure hospital staff working with severe malaria patients have adequate knowledge and skills – to ensure equipment and supplies for malaria in all district hospitals	– 90% of staff meet skills criteria for severe malaria as laid down in national guidelines – all district hospitals have all equipment listed in national guidelines functional for at least 300 days per year – stock-outs of supplies for severe malaria as prescribed in national guidelines reduced to no more that ten days per year
One-year objectives: – to design and initiate a staff development programme for severe malaria – to conduct a needs assessment and survey of equipment and supplies for severe malaria in the district, and initiate a programme for improvement	– programme developed and first module completed and appraised in two hospitals by year end – needs assessment and survey completed, and detailed plan for improvement completed by year end

Plan activities

Once priorities and objectives have been identified, the next step is a detailed work plan and budget. Planning and budgeting for activities is often cyclical: once you have detailed plans, you may need to refine the budget. If all the resources needed are not available, you may then need to modify the plan to bring it within budget. It may be helpful to identify potential funding sources early in the process of planning. It will also be useful to find out what kind of activities the funds can be used for and the mechanisms for applying, so that proposals can be submitted at an early stage.

At district and sub-district level it will generally make more sense to structure plans and budgets in terms of the level of service (community, first-line health facilities, higher level health centres, hospitals, referral hospitals, etc.) rather than in terms of individual diseases. It may then be important to ensure that objectives, activities and resources at each level reflect the burden of malaria. For example, for lower level health unit services:

• Do plans for procuring and managing drugs include enough anti-malarial drugs for malaria case management, including pre-referral treatment?
• Do staff training plans include adequate malaria case management training, as well as adequate training in advising on preventive measures such as insecticide-treated mosquito nets?
• Do staff have skills and resources for community mobilisation for malaria prevention and early care seeking?

Formats for work plans vary, and there may be local or national guidelines. Generally for each activity they specify the action, who is responsible, who else is involved, the budget, the timescale (start and end dates) and sometimes 'milestones'.

Detailed work plans should include activities for the next stages in the planning cycle, for example mobilising resources, supervision activities and monitoring and evaluation.

Finally, how often do you need to plan? Planning is a continuous process. Plans need to be reviewed regularly in the light of available resources, progress being made (see Monitoring and evaluation below), and unexpected developments (for example, a sudden policy change or unusual weather which affects the incidence of malaria).

Reorganise and mobilise/Implement – putting plans into action

'Selling' the plan

Depending on how different the new plan is from what is currently being done, the first stages of implementation may involve 'selling' the plan, particularly to those affected by or involved in the change (especially if there are major changes), to the people who allocate resources (financial and human resources, equipment, etc.) within the district, and to other potential funding sources.

For example, assume that the district wants to achieve better compliance with recommended drug regimes in order to reduce mortality. Clearly more will be achieved if community members, health workers, supervisors and trainers recognise the need and want to do something about it. If as many of these people as possible were involved at the planning stage, they will have more confidence that this is the right way forward, be motivated to act, and be more likely feel accountable for their actions.

Even then, complete agreement is rare, so skills in persuasion and motivation will be very important at this stage. Managing change is an important skill and is covered in many texts.

Getting people and systems in place

Once there is good support for the plan, the necessary components must be set in place – people, materials, systems. For example, it may be necessary to recruit new people and retrain existing staff, negotiate with partners on activities they might do on your behalf, reorganise teams and the space in which they work. You may need to buy new equipment and ensure that supplies of materials, salary payments and care of equipment run smoothly. Here, people with logistical skills will have an important role.

Training often features heavily at the early stages of implementation. It is certainly important, but it is usually not enough on its own. Elements such as clear allocation of duties, adequate materials, good support from supervisors, reward for improved performance, and clear lines of accountability are also important.

Supervision

Once implementation is underway, good supervision – to develop and motivate staff and keep work on track – is vital. There may

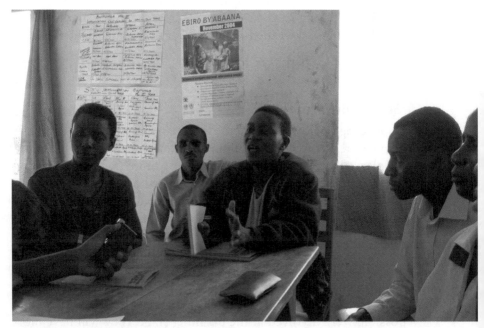

Figure 7.2: Inviting feedback is important in supervision: malaria volunteers describe their work in Uganda

be national or local supervision guidelines and this chapter does not attempt to cover good supervision practice in any detail. It is likely that supervision at lower levels of health service will cover much more than just malaria. While it is useful to have checklists for supervision, it is also important that supervisors are responsive to the concerns and problems of the people being supervised – and that the supervisors themselves have sources of support and professional guidance from peers and line managers.

Monitoring and evaluation

The definition of Monitoring & Evaluation (M&E) used here is given in Box 7.5.

Box 7.5: Monitoring and evaluation

Monitoring is a systematic process to assess the progress of ongoing activities as planned and identify problems and constraints so they can be quickly corrected.

Evaluation is a systematic process of measuring effectiveness and efficiency of the desired objectives or outcomes of the work.

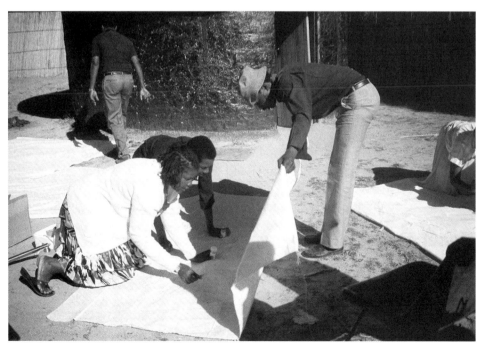

Figure 7.3: A pyrethrum spray catch to count the number of mosquitoes resting in a house in order to evaluate the vector control programme in Namibia

Malaria presents many challenges for monitoring and evaluation. It is difficult to distinguish malaria from other fevers where resources for diagnosis are limited. Many cases of malaria never come to health facilities, interventions are often community based, and their impact cannot be easily or cheaply measured. However, provided the objectives have 'SMART' targets or indicators (see Box 7.6), it should be possible to identify how you are going to monitor progress against your plan and to evaluate how well objectives and outputs are being achieved.

Box 7.6: 'SMART' targets and indicators

SMART = **S**pecific, **M**easurable, **A**ppropriate, **R**ealistic and **T**ime-bound

Example of a SMART indicator:

'To increase the number of health facilities with adequate parasite detection services from seven to ten by year aaaa, according to national policy'

- This is *specific* – its meaning should be clear to most people and 'adequate' will be defined by what the national policy says.
- It is *measurable* – you can count the facilities that meet policy requirements.
- It is *appropriate* – it relates to policy.
- It is *realistic* – it can be achieved, provided the resources are there.
- It is *time-bound* – it must be done by year aaaa.

Monitoring and evaluation requires a system for collecting, analysing, reporting and acting on information that will tell you something about progress being made and its effectiveness. Managers may want to monitor how many people are trained to the necessary standard (output) and also the resources that go into the activity (input), how it is managed (process), and the effect on the quality of case management (impact). An example is given below.

Model example

It is January 2006 in Goodhealth District. The District Health Team's work plan for the year August 2005 to July 2006 has had as one of its objectives: 'by July 2006, to train at least 120 health care workers at first-level facilities on national guidelines for case management of uncomplicated malaria'. Four monitoring indicators were selected.

The detailed plan was that one training course would be held every three months, each covering at least 30 staff. The budget was $1500 per workshop or $50 per student, covering all costs apart from staff time. Five trainers (one national and four district) were to be deployed, each devoting one day for preparation for each course, four days for the training course itself and one day per month for monitoring and follow-up. In addition, a secretary was deployed for three days for each workshop to help with organisation and paperwork.

Table 7.1 shows the monitoring methodology used and the monitoring results submitted by the training team to the District Director of Health Services in October 2005.

On receiving the monitoring report, the DDHS congratulated the training team on completing their first course and on their constructive proposals for dealing with problems that the monitoring had highlighted. He endorsed all these except for the increase in budget. He asked the team to come up with proposals for enhancing the course content within the existing budget, as there was no additional money available. He also recommended that the health workers who had done less well should receive more help through longer follow-up visits. Those who had done better should still be visited regularly, but were likely to need less time.

The team accepted these recommendations and later came back with a proposal, which the DDHS endorsed, to extend the course within the existing budget by adding an extra 30 minutes a day to the timetable and sending participants materials to read beforehand. The subsequent course was attended by 33 staff. Average scores were 3/10 before the course and 9/10 after, compared with 3/10 and 7/10 respectively in the first course.

Comment   This example is designed to illustrate the benefits of monitoring to those who are closely involved in the work (in this instance, the training team). These benefits include:

▶ spotting problems early and dealing with them to bring the task back on track
▶ solving your own problems – having ownership of the task
▶ learning by doing and feeding this back into future planning
▶ improving communication within the team and with the boss.

It also illustrates aspects of good management on the boss's part: praising good work, giving constructive criticism where improvement is needed, and encouraging staff to generate ideas.

Table 7.1 Monitoring of malaria case management training in Goodhealth District

Objective: By July 2006, to train at least 120 health care workers at first-level facilities on national guidelines for case management of uncomplicated malaria

	Indicator	Methodology	Position at October 2005	Analysis	Recommendation from team
Impact	% of cases managed correctly according to guidelines before and after training	One of the trainers observed management of one case by each course participant immediately before and one month after the training, using a checklist to establish whether they did ten essential things correctly	Before – average score 3/10 After – average score 7/10	Definite improvement following training – persistent mistakes were mainly due to the missing elements on the training course, but there was inadequate counselling of the patient or carer	We propose to spend more time on counselling skills next time and amend the handouts to cover this aspect more thoroughly.
Output	Number of workers trained by agreed methodology	One of the trainers examined on attendance records, and workshop programmes and reports A quality assurance report from a national supervisor who visited the training for half a day	25 health workers trained Two aspects of case management were not covered adequately	The omissions were mainly due to the absence of one trainer Five workers failed to attend for unknown reasons	We need a reserve trainer in case of unavoidable absence and to cover for each other better We shall ensure these five health workers attend next time and increase the size of the group to make up

	Indicator	Methodology	Position at October 2005	Analysis	Recommendation from team
Process	Number invited to each training course	The secretary kept invitation letters on file	30 health workers were invited to the course	This was as originally planned but leaves no leeway	We shall invite more next time to allow for some non-attenders
Input	Cost per workshop and per person trained, number of days spent by trainers on training	Examination of accounts records, workshop reports and checking with individual trainers	This first workshop cost $1000 or $40 per person The national trainer and three district trainers gave the necessary time One of the trainers spent one day on preparation but missed the course due to sickness	The lower cost was due to the lower attendance, the absence of one trainer and some savings on transport	We shall use the savings to allow higher attendance next time. In addition we recommend a budget increase, so we can lengthen the course by one day

Key points

> ► Good management makes a huge difference to the success of health services, malaria control included.
>
> ► Good planning is the basis for good management and should feature:
>   - the involvement of key stakeholders during the process
>   - a shared vision of where you want to be in the longer term
>   - the collection of relevant information
>   - a process of assessing information in order to identify clear and achievable objectives and outputs
>   - a realistic view of available resources and good knowledge about funding sources.
>
> ► Successful implementation requires:
>   - maintaining the shared vision
>   - clarity on objectives, responsibilities and lines of accountability
>   - effective change management skills
>   - establishing the right environment for success: having the people, funds, systems and infrastructure in place and well organised
>   - ongoing supportive supervision and professional development
>   - ongoing monitoring and **feedback** into the plan.
>
> ► Planning and implementation are dynamic processes and benefit from regular review and amendment in the light of progress, resources available, changes in the external environment and lessons learned.

Further reading

'Current challenges in malaria' (p4 'Planning for malaria control') *Health Action*, Issue 26, May–August 2000

Glossary

A

Abdomen: (human) the portion of the body which lies between the thorax and the pelvis.

Abdomen: (insect) the hindmost of the three segments into which insects' bodies are divided.

Access: the right and the ability to obtain or make use of a service or facility.

Acidaemia: a blood disorder caused by an increase in the hydrogen-ion concentration of the blood or a fall below normal on the pH scale.

Active surveillance: (see **surveillance, active**)

Adherence: following the recommendations of a doctor, other health care provider, or investigator in a research project.

Agranulocytosis: a condition in which there is an insufficient number of white blood cells called neutrophils or *granulocytes*.

Algorithm: a process consisting of steps, each depending on the outcome of the previous one. In clinical medicine, a step-by-step protocol for management of a health care problem.

Anaemia: a reduction in the quantity of the oxygen-carrying pigment 'haemoglobin' in the blood. The main symptoms are tiredness, breathlessness on exertion, pallor, and poor resistance to infection.

Anopheles: the genus of mosquito which is host to the malaria parasite (*Plasmodium*) and which transmits the parasite to humans.

Antennae: the pair of large sense organs which are rooted between a mosquito's eyes – they are very bushy in males and much less so in females.

Annual parasite index: the number of parasitologically confirmed malaria cases per a given number, usually 1,000 persons per year.

Antigen/antigenic: any substance which the body recognises as foreign or toxic and therefore triggers an immune response.

Anti-malarial: a drug used to prevent or treat malaria.

Asymptomatic: not showing any symptoms, whether disease is present or not (see **parasitaemia**).

B

Basic case reproduction rate: a measure of the potential number of new cases of malaria that will result from any one case.

Bendiocarb: one of the carbamate insecticides frequently used for indoor residual spraying.

Bias: any trend in the collection, analysis, interpretation, publication, or review of data that can lead to conclusions that are systematically different from the truth.

Blood meal: blood ingested by a female mosquito from a vertebrate host.

Breeding site (place): site where eggs, larvae or pupae of mosquitoes are found; larval habitat.

Bruxism: involuntary grinding of the teeth.

Buccal mucous: mucous in buccal glands in the submucous tissue of the cheeks.

C

Capacity: the resources people possess, mobilise or have access to that allow them to have control over shaping their own futures. Resources may be physical assets (land, money), skills (literacy, technical), social situation (community organisation), personal characteristics (will to survive), or beliefs (religion).

Carbamate: pesticide with a chemical structure related to carbamic acid.

Case: a person who has the particular disease, health disorder, or condition which meets the case definitions for surveillance and outbreak investigation purposes. The definition of a case for surveillance and outbreak investigation is not necessarily the same as the ordinary clinical definition.

Case definition: a set of diagnostic criteria that must be fulfilled for an individual to be regarded as a case of a particular disease for surveillance or outbreak investigation purposes. Case definitions can be based on clinical criteria, laboratory criteria or a combination of both.

Case detection: one of the activities of surveillance operations concerned with the continuous search for new cases in a community.

Cerebral malaria: impairment of consciousness in a patient with *Plasmodium falciparum* malaria (definition often confined to cases with unrousable coma).

Cell: the smallest unit of a living structure capable of independent existence.

Chemoprophylaxis: the administration of a chemical, to prevent the development of an infection or the progression of an infection to active manifest disease.

Coma: a state of profound unconsciousness from which the individual cannot be roused.

Community: a group of individuals living together in some form of social organisation with cohesion in planning and operation. In health care organisation, it refers to the most local level of the health system.

Community health worker (CHW): a member of the community who is integrated into primary health care programmes after short training on health-related issues and acts as an intermediary between the community and health services. CHWs may be recruited as paid staff or volunteers (CHVs).

Community participation: occurs when communities, rather than being just beneficiaries of health care, share the responsibility of caring for their health.

Compliance: (see **adherence**)

Convulsion: a violent spasm or involuntary contracting of the muscles. Also known as a seizure.

Coverage: a measure of the extent to which services cover the potential need for these services in a community. It is expressed as a proportion in which the numerator is the number of services rendered and the denominator is the number of instances in which the service should have been rendered.

Crepitations: crackling or rattling sound (rale).

Cure, clinical: relief of symptoms (e.g. by chemotherapeutic action, against asexual erythrocytic parasites) without complete elimination of the infection.

Cure, radical: complete elimination of the (malaria) parasite from the body so that relapses cannot occur. Radical cure may be brought about by natural means in the absence of specific medication (natural or spontaneous cure), by radical treatment, or by suppressive cure.

Cyanosis: a bluish or purplish discolouring (of skin, nailbeds, lips) due to deficient oxygenation of the blood.

Cytoplasm: the living matter within a cell (apart from the nucleus) that causes the cell to function.

D

Data: a collection of items of information.

Death rate (Mortality rate): the number of deaths in a group of people in a given period of time (most often expressed as deaths per thousand per year).

Deltamethrin: one of the pyrethroid insecticides which is widely used to treat mosquito nets and for indoor residual spraying.

Demography: the statistical study of human populations, especially with reference to size and density, distribution and vital statistics.

Denominator: the bottom number in a fraction used to calculate a rate or ratio. In health terms, the population (or population experience, in person-years) at risk in the calculation of a rate or ratio.

DDT (dichlorodiphenyltrichloroethane): one of the organochlorine insecticides which has been widely used for indoor residual spraying.

Differential diagnosis: a systematic method of determining the particular disease an individual is suffering from when the disease has symptoms that are not unique.

District: the smallest defined administrative and operational unit of government.

District hospitals: health facilities which provide in- and out-patient services (usually referred from community health centres or clinics) but with medical services usually limited to emergency obstetrical and surgical care and follow up, in-patient and rehabilitative care. Facilities include laboratory, blood bank, and X-ray services.

Dose, loading: an initial dose of a drug which is higher than that regularly used.

E

Early warning system: a system which monitors indicators to facilitate the early identification of potential epidemic situations.

Effectiveness: a measure of the extent to which a specific intervention, procedure, regimen, or service, when deployed in the field in routine circumstances, does what it is intended to do for a specified population. In the health field, it is a measure of output from those health services that contribute towards reducing the dimension of a problem or improving an unsatisfactory situation.

Efficacy: the extent to which a specific intervention, procedure, regimen, or service produces a beneficial result under ideal conditions.

Efficiency: the effects or end results achieved in relation to the effort expended in terms of money, resources and time; the extent to which the resources used to provide a specific intervention, procedure, regimen, or service of known efficacy and effectiveness are minimised.

Endemic: the continuous or regular presence of a disease or infectious agent within a given geographical area or a population group.

Endemicity, malaria: the intensity of malaria transmission in a given area, usually measured by malaria surveys.

Epidemic: The occurrence of more cases of disease than expected in a given area or among a specific group of people over a particular period of time. The community or region and the period in which the cases occur are specified precisely. The number of cases indicating the presence of an epidemic varies according to the agent, size, and type of population exposed, previous experience or lack of exposure to the disease, and time and place of occurrence.

Epidemic curve: A graphic plotting of the distribution of cases by time of onset.

Epidemiology: The study of the distribution and determinants of health-related states or events in specified populations, and the application of this study to control of health problems.

Erythrocyte: a mature red blood cell.

Essential drugs: (also essential medicines) are defined by WHO as those that satisfy the priority health care needs of the population. They should be available within the context of functioning health systems at all times in adequate amounts, in the appropriate dosage forms, with assured quality, and at a price the individual and the community can afford.

Evaluation: a process that attempts to determine as systematically and objectively as possible the relevance, effectiveness, and impact of activities in the light of their objectives. Different types of evaluation can be distinguished, e.g. evaluation of structure, process, and outcomes.

Exflagellation: the stage in the life cycle of the malaria parasite when the male gametocyte is activated in the mosquito stomach. The gametocyte forms into eight nuclei from which long thread-like flagella form, then break out of the gametocyte.

Exo-erythrocytic: stage in the life cycle of the malaria parasite in the liver of the vertebrate host before the erythrocytic phase in the red blood cells (erythrocytes).

Extrinsic incubation period: time it takes for a disease agent to develop in a vector – i.e. the time from the uptake of the agent to the time when the vector becomes infective.

F

Febrile: feverish or related to fever.

Feedback: the transmission of evaluation findings to parties for whom it is relevant and useful to help increase knowledge. It may involve the collection and dissemination of findings, conclusions, recommendations and lessons learnt from experience.

Fenitrothion: one of the organophosphate insecticides used for indoor residual spraying.

Flagellum: the form of the male gamete – a long thread-like structure which is formed from the nuclei of the male gametocyte (see exflagellation).

Focus groups: a group of individuals chosen to discuss the topic that is the subject of the research.

Follow-up: observation over a period of time of an individual, group, or initially defined population, whose relevant characteristics have been assessed in order to observe changes in health status or health-related variables.

Fontanelle: a membranous space in an infant's skull.

G

Gamete: mature sexual form, male or female. In malaria parasites the female gametes (macrogametes) and the male gametes (microgametes) normally develop in the mosquito.

Gametocytes: parent cell of a gamete. In malaria parasites, the female gametocytes (macrogametocytes) and the male gametocytes (microgametocytes) develop in the red blood cell. Very young gametocytes cannot usually be distinguished from trophozoites.

Going to scale: the replication of a pilot scheme to national or regional scale.

Gonotrophic cycle: one complete round of ovarian development in the mosquito from the time when the blood meal is taken to the time when the fully developed eggs are laid.

H

Haematocrit: the ratio of the volume occupied by packed red blood cells after centrifugation to the volume of the whole blood or the name of the instrument used to take this measurement.

Haemoglobin: a protein containing iron in the red blood cells that carries oxygen (and makes the blood red).

Haemoglobinopathy: a genetic disease affecting haemoglobin, e.g. sickle cell anaemia.

Haemoglobinuria: the presence of haemoglobin in the urine.

Haemolysis: the destruction of red blood cells.

Haemorrhage: the escape of blood from a vessel.

Health centre: a facility providing primary health care, usually at community level.

Health education: the process by which individuals and groups of people learn to behave in a manner conducive to the promotion, maintenance, or restoration of health.

Hepatic: relating to the liver.

Hepatocyte: a liver cell.

Hepatomegaly: enlargement of the liver.

Holoendemic: perennial high level transmission of malaria resulting in a considerable degree of immune response in all age groups, particularly in adults.

Hookworm: one of the intestinal parasites which is an important cause of anaemia.

Host: a human or other animal that nourishes and supports a parasite. A transport host is a carrier for an infectious agent. In an epidemiological context, the host may be the population or group; biological, social, and behavioural characteristics of this group that are relevant to health are called 'host factors'.

Household: the people who occupy a single housing unit – not necessarily related to one another.

Hyperendemic: intense but seasonal transmission where the immunity is insufficient to prevent the effects of malaria on all age groups.

Hyperpyrexia: extremely high fever.

Hypersensitive: showing an excessive immune response to the presence of a particular antigen.

Hypnozoite: dormant form of the *P. vivax* and *P. ovale* malaria parasite which remains in the liver and may cause relapses.

Hypoendemic: low malaria transmission where its effect on the general population is of low significance.

Hypoglycaemia: an abnormally small concentration of glucose in the blood.

Hypotension: low blood pressure.

I

Immunisation (vaccination): the process of inducing immunity to communicable disease in a susceptible individual by the administration of a living modified agent (as in yellow fever), a suspension of killed organisms (as in whooping cough), or an inactivated toxin (as in tetanus).

Immunity, acquired: resistance acquired by a host as a result of previous exposure to a natural pathogen or substance that is foreign to the host.

Implementation: in development terms 'the process of realising a project 'on the ground' in line with the agreed work plan. It involves Project Management and Monitoring – both financial and non-financial.'

Incubation period: the time from contact with infectious agents (bacteria, viruses, fungi, or parasites) to onset of disease.

Incidence: the number of new cases of a disease that develop within a specified population over a specified period of time.

Incidence rate: a measure of the frequency with which new cases of an illness occur in a population. The numerator is the number of new events that occur in a defined period and the denominator is the population at risk of experiencing the event during this period, sometimes expressed as person-time.

Indicator: a measure that shows whether a standard has been reached. It is used to measure and communicate the results of programmes as well as the process or methods used. Indicators can be qualitative or quantitative.

Infection, mixed: malaria infection with more than one species of *Plasmodium*.

Integrated Management of Childhood Illness (IMCI): a system of diagnosing and treating childhood illnesses based on assessment of clinical symptoms.

Intermittent preventive treatment (IPT): the use of anti-malarial drugs during pregnancy given at treatment doses (preferably single dose) at predefined intervals after 'quickening' (first noted foetal movement by the mother) to reduce the consequences of malaria infection.

Internally displaced persons: people who have been forced to leave their homes suddenly or unexpectedly in large numbers, as a result of armed conflict, internal strife, systematic violations of human rights, or natural or man-made disasters, and who are within the territory of their own country.

K

Koplik spots: small red spots on the buccal mucous membrane.

L

Lambdacyhalothrin: one of the pyrethroid insecticides used both for indoor residual spraying and for mosquito net treatment.

Larva: The pre-adult or immature stage hatching from the egg of some animal groups, e.g. insects and nematodes, which may be markedly different from the sexually mature adult and have a totally different way of life. In the case of *Anopheles* the larvae live in fairly clean water and float parallel to the surface.

Logistics: The procurement, distribution, maintenance and replacement of material and personnel.

M

Macrogamete: (see **gamete**)

Malathion: one of the organophosphate insecticides used for indoor residual spraying.

Man-biting habit: the number of times per day that the mosquito feeds on humans. For a highly anthropophilic mosquito, such as *Anopheles gambiae*, with a gonotrophic cycle lasting two or three days, the value for the 'man-biting habit' would be 0.33 to 0.5.

Merozoite: a stage in the life cycle of the malaria parasite. Many merozoites are formed during the asexual division of the schizont. The released merozoites may invade new red blood cells or new liver cells, and continue the asexual phase with the production of yet more merozoites, effectively spreading the infection. Alternatively, merozoites invade red blood cells and begin the sexual cycle with the formation of male and female gametocytes.

Mesoendemic: moderate levels of transmission intensity, typically found among small rural communities in the sub-tropical zones.

Microgamete: (see **gamete**)

Monitoring: episodic measurement of the effect of an intervention on the health status of a population or environment. The process of collecting and analysing information about the implementation of a programme for the purpose of identifying problems, such as non-compliance, and taking corrective action. Not to be confused with surveillance, although the techniques of surveillance may be used in monitoring. In management, the episodic oversight of the implementation of an activity, seeking to ensure that inputs, deliveries, work schedules, targeted outputs, and other required actions are proceeding according to plan.

Morbidity: any departure, subjective or objective, from a state of physiological or psychological well-being. In this sense *sickness*, *illness* and *morbid condition* are similarly defined and synonymous. Morbidity could be measured in terms of three units: (a) people who are ill; (b) the illnesses that these people experience; and (c) the duration of these illnesses.

Mortality rate: (see **death rate**)

Multigravida: a pregnant woman who has had previous pregnancies.

Myalgia: pain in the muscles.

N

Needs assessment: A systematic procedure for determining the nature and extent of problems experienced by a specified population, that affect their health either directly or indirectly. Needs assessment makes use of epidemiological, socio-demographic and qualitative methods to describe health problems and their environmental, social, economic, and behavioural determinants. The aim is to identify unmet health care needs and make recommendations about ways to address these needs.

Normocytic: any anaemia in which the erythrocytes are normal in size.

Nystagmus: involuntary rapid movement of the eyes.

O

Oedema: swelling caused by too much fluid in the tissues.

Oliguria: the production of an abnormally small amount of urine.

Organochlorine: a synthetically produced organic compound containing chlorine and used as an insecticide, e.g. DDT, dieldrin.

Organophosphate: a category of insecticide whose molecules may be derived from phosphoric and similar acids, and which interferes with an insect's nervous system.

Otitis media: inflammation of the middle ear.

Outbreak: an epidemic limited to a localised increase in the incidence of a disease, e.g. in a village, town or closed institution.

Outcomes: all the possible results that may stem from exposure to a causal factor or from preventive or therapeutic interventions; all identified changes in health status arising as a consequence of the handling of a health problem.

P

Pallor: paleness, paler or lighter than normal.

Palmar: relating to the palms (fronts) of the hands.

Palps: the pair of sense organs rooted just above the proboscis of mosquitoes – they are as long as the proboscis in female *Anopheles* mosquitoes and very short in female culicine mosquitoes – this difference is the most conclusive way of telling female *Anopheles* (malaria vectors) apart from other types of female mosquito.

Parasitaemia: the presence of parasites in the blood (used especially with reference to malarial and other protozoan forms of parasite – and also used as a synonym for parasite density).

Parasite: An animal or vegetable organism that lives on or in and derives its nourishment from another organism.

Parasite clearance time: time elapsing from the first drug administration to the first occasion on which no parasites can be seen in the blood.

Parasite count: number of parasites per micro litre of blood on a given slide.

Parasite density: the number of parasites per unit volume of blood (see **parasitaemia**).

Parasite rate: the percentage of people who have a positive blood slide test for malaria parasite.

Participatory rural appraisal: a technique used for gathering information about rural conditions and people, which involves the local people.

Passive surveillance: (see **surveillance, passive**)

Parenteral: administered directly into the blood system rather than through the mouth, e.g by injection.

Participation: the involvement of the community in the decision-making process.

Perinatal: just before or just after birth.

Pirimiphos-methyl: one of the organophosphate insecticides used for indoor residual spraying.

Plasmodium: generic name of the parasites that cause malaria in humans and other organisms.

Postural hypotension: low blood pressure occurring in some people when they stand up.

Prevalence: the number of cases in a given population affected with a particular disease or condition at a given time – c.f. incidence which is the number of new cases per unit of time.

Prevention: activities aimed at minimising the impact of disease and defined as three levels: primary, secondary and tertiary. Primary prevention is an active assertive process of creating conditions (e.g. by vaccination, chemoprophylaxis or vector control) and/or personal attributes that promotes the well being of people. Secondary prevention is early detection and intervention to keep beginning problems from becoming more severe.

Primigravida: a woman who is pregnant for the first time.

Proboscis: the feeding tube of certain insects, e.g. female mosquitoes where its complex structure includes tubes for the inward passage of blood and the outward passage of saliva (which may contain *Plasmodium* sporozoites.

Prophylaxis: (see **chemoprophylaxis**)

Prostration: extreme exhaustion, loss of strength.

Protocol: the plan, or series of steps, to be followed in a study or investigation or in an intervention programme.

Puerperal: relating to the period immediately after childbirth.

Pulmonary: relating to, associated with or affecting the lungs.

Pulmonary oedema: a build up of fluid in the lungs.

Pyelonephritis: inflammation of the drainage system of the kidneys.

Pyrethroid: the category of synthetic chemical insecticides which are similar to the natural chemical pyrethrum.

R

Random sample: a sample in which each individual in a population has the same chance of being selected as any other.

Rapid appraisal: an assessment of the impact of a policy, a programme or a situation using minimal resources in a short time frame.

Rate: a measure of the frequency with which an event occurs in a defined population in a specified period of time. The use of rates rather than raw numbers is essential for comparison of experience between populations at different times, different places, or of different classes. The components of a rate are the numerator, the denominator, the specified time in which events occur, and usually a multiplier, a power of 10, that converts the rate from an awkward fraction or decimal to a whole number.

$$\text{Rate} = \frac{\text{Number of events in specified period} \times 10^n}{\text{Average population during the period}}$$

The word 'rate' may also be used for prevalence of certain conditions at a given point or period of time, e.g. spleen rate.

Ratio: the relationship in quantity, amount or size between two or more things. (e.g. if the ratio of chickens to goats is 10:2 and there are 20 chickens, there will be 4 goats).

Recrudescence: renewed manifestation of infection after a period of latency following the primary attack. It is particularly used to describe treatment failure of *Plasmodium falciparum* and needs to be distinguished from a new infection due to a new mosquito bite.

Refugee: Someone who has fled his or her country because he/she has a 'well-founded fear of persecution for reasons of race, religion, nationality, membership in a particular social group or political opinion' (definition used by United Nations).

Relapse: recurrence of a disease after an initial response to treatment. In relation specifically to malaria, the renewed manifestation (of clinical symptoms and/or parasitaemia) of malaria infection separated from previous manifestations of the same infection by an interval greater than those due to the normal cycle of symptoms. The term is used mainly for renewed manifestation due to survival of exo-erythrocytic forms of *Plasmodium vivax* or *P. ovale.*

Relative humidity: the amount of water vapour in the air, compared to the amount the air could hold if it was totally saturated.

Resistance: the ability of a parasite (or insect) strain to multiply or to survive in the presence of concentrations of a drug (or insecticide) that normally destroy parasites or insects of the same species or prevent their multiplication.

Rigors: shaking or shivering of the body (especially as a symptom of malaria).

Risk: the probability that an event will occur, e.g. that an individual will become ill or die within a stated period of time or by a certain age. Also a non-technical term encompassing a variety of measures of the probability of an unfavourable outcome.

S

Sample: a selected sub-set of a population. A sample may be random or non-random and may be representative or non-representative.

Schizogony: the asexual phase of the life cycle of the human malaria parasite.

Schizont: intracellular asexual form of the malaria parasite, developing either in tissue or in blood cells.

Seasonal transmission: when transmission occurs only during some months and is totally interrupted or very low during other months.

Sentinel surveillance: surveillance based on selected population samples chosen to represent the relevant experience of particular groups. Mosquito sampling may also be conducted at regular intervals in 'sentinel houses' to represent a whole vaillage.

Sepsis: the presence of pathogenic bacteria in the blood.

Signs and symptoms: 'sign' refers to objective evidence of disease. A sign can be detected by a person other than the affected individual. For example, a bloody nose is a sign of disease. It can be recognised by the patient, doctor, nurse or others.

A **symptom** is subjective. Abdominal pain is a symptom. It is something only the patient can know. Anxiety, lower back pain, and fatigue are all symptoms. They are sensations only the patient can perceive.

Situation analysis: an analysis carried out to understand the problems and needs of a specific group of people in a specific setting. It can use a variety of data-gathering techniques and assess a variety of perspectives (social, economic, environmental).

Species: group of organisms capable of exchanging genetic material with one another and incapable, because of their genetic constitution, of exchanging such material with any other group of organisms.

Spleen rate: a term used in malaria epidemiology to define the prevalence of enlarged spleens detected on survey of a population in which malaria is prevalent. In association with the Hackett Spleen Classification, it summarises the extent of malaria endemicity.

Splenomegaly: enlarged spleen.

Sporozoite: the infective form of the malaria parasite occurring either in a mature oocyst before its rupture or in the salivary glands of the mosquito.

Sporogony: the sexual phase of the life cycle of the human malaria parasite i.e. from when a mosquito imbibes gametocytes to when infective sporozoites are produced.

Stable malaria: stable transmission areas are those where there is a steady prevalence which does not show great change during a transmission season or from one season to another, except as a result of extreme changes in environmental factors. Epidemics are unlikely and the affected population often shows a high level of immunity.

Stakeholder analysis: an analysis of the people and/or groups of people who need to be considered when planning policy or programmes.

Stakeholder: any individual or group that may be affected by, or may influence, a policy, programme or intervention.

Standard: a basis for comparison against which other things can be evaluated.

Sternum: the breastbone.

Surveillance: in health terms, the systematic collection, analysis, interpretation, and dissemination of health data on an ongoing basis, to gain knowledge of the pattern of disease occurrence and potential in a community, in order to control and prevent disease in the community.

Surveillance may be **active** in which those making the survey take the initiative and seek out members of the community from which to take samples or measurements. Alternatively surveillance may be **passive** in which members of the community who feel ill take the initiative by going to a health facility where data are collected.

Survey: an investigation in which information is systematically collected. Usually carried out in a sample of a defined population group, within a defined time period. Unlike surveillance it is not ongoing. However, if repeated regularly, surveys can form the basis of a surveillance system.

Symptoms: (see **signs and symptoms**)

T

Tachycardia: rapid beating of the heart.

Tachypnoea: rapid breathing.

Target population: the group of people you are trying to reach with a particular strategy or activity.

Temephos: one of the organophosphate insecticides which is widely used against mosquito larvae (trade name: 'Abate').

Transmission: any mechanism by which an infectious agent is spread from a source or reservoir to another person.

Trophozoite: In malaria terminology, generally used to indicate intracellular erythrocytic forms in their early stages of development. Trophozoites may be in either a ring stage or an early amoeboid or solid stage, but always have the nucleus still undivided.

U

Unstable malaria: unstable transmission areas are those where one or more conditions necessary for the transmission of malaria are missing – if and when these appear the transmission rate can change suddenly and significantly.

V

Vector: an insect or any living carrier that transports an infectious agent from an infected individual or its wastes to a susceptible individual or its food or immediate surroundings. The organism may or may not pass though a developmental cycle within the vector. In the case of malaria *Anopheles* mosquitoes are the vectors.

Vector control: measures of any kind directed against a vector of disease and intended to reduce disease transmission.

Vectorial capacity: the capacity of a vector (mosquito) population to transmit malaria in a given area. As expressed by Macdonald's equation.

$$\text{Vectorial capacity} = \frac{ma^2p^n}{-\log_e p}$$

where m = the population of mosquitoes relative to that of humans
       a = man biting habit (qv)
       n = duration of sporogony (qv)
       p = probability of a mosquito surviving to the next day

Vulnerability: defencelessness, insecurity and exposure to risks. In development terms, 'the propensity of a population group to experience substantial damage, disruption and casualties as a result of a hazard'.

Sources

Cogsci.princeton.edu (Lexical Database, Cognitive Science Laboratory, Princeton)

Concise medical dictionary, fifth edition, 1998, Oxford University Press

IIME (Institute of International Medical Education) Glossary of Medical Education Terms, http://www.iime.org/glossary.htm

Last, J. *A dictionary of epidemiology*, fourth edition, 2001, Oxford University Press

Stedman's Concise Medical Dictionary for the Health Professions, fourth edition, 2001, Lippincott, Williams and Wilkins

Slee, V *et al. Health care terms*, third edition, 1996, Saint Paul, Minn. Tringa Press

Index